EMPOWERING YOUR LIFE WITH
YOGA

EMPOWERING YOUR LIFE WITH
YOGA

Bliss Wood

ALPHA

A member of Penguin Group (USA) Inc.

To every student who has become my teacher—to every teacher I have yet to meet—and to all of you, with whom I share in this great journey ... I honor you!

International Standard Book Number: 1-59257-249-9
Library of Congress Catalog Card Number: 2004103239

06   05   04   8   7   6   5   4   3   2   1

Interpretation of the printing code: The rightmost number of the first series of numbers is the year of the book's printing; the rightmost number of the second series of numbers is the number of the book's printing. For example, a printing code of 04-1 shows that the first printing occurred in 2004.

Printed in the United States of America

Note: This publication contains the opinions and ideas of its author. It is intended to provide helpful and informative material on the subject matter covered. It is sold with the understanding that the author and publisher are not engaged in rendering professional services in the book. If the reader requires personal assistance or advice, a competent professional should be consulted.

The author and publisher specifically disclaim any responsibility for any liability, loss, or risk, personal or otherwise, which is incurred as a consequence, directly or indirectly, of the use and application of any of the contents of this book.

Most Alpha books are available at special quantity discounts for bulk purchases for sales promotions, premiums, fund-raising, or educational use. Special books, or book excerpts, can also be created to fit specific needs.

For details, write: Special Markets, Alpha Books, 375 Hudson Street, New York, NY 10014.

Publisher: Marie Butler-Knight
Product Manager: Phil Kitchel
Senior Managing Editor: Jennifer Chisholm
Acquisitions Editor: Mikal Belicove
Development Editor: Lynn Northrup
Senior Production Editor: Billy Fields
Copy Editor: Sara Fink
Cover Designers: Charis Santille, Doug Wilkins
Book Designer: Trina Wurst
Creative Director: Robin Lasek
Indexer: Angie Bess
Layout/Proofreading: John Etchison, Becky Harmon

Contents

Introduction

Yoga is an ancient tradition that subscribes to no religion. It began in India more than 5,000 years ago and was used as a tool to help yogis reach nirvana. Today, the ultimate goal of yoga is still to reach nirvana; however, in this modern age of high technology and "bigger is better," we have found yoga to be an empowerment tool on a regular basis. Its positive effects can be seen and felt every day through deeper relationships, more focused career paths, and a simpler, more honest way of communicating with ourselves and others.

Yoga combines spiritual traditions, physical movements, and a philosophy of life that leads to enlightenment. Yoga deepens our spirituality, and matures our attitudes and intentions toward life by integrating body, mind, and spirit.

The word *yoga* comes from the Sanskrit term meaning "union" or "yoke." Therefore, the practice of yoga seeks to create unity between the mind, body, and spirit of a person. We'll become less fragmented inwardly and become more comfortable in our own skin, developing greater self-confidence, inner strength, and a profound peace that overflows from our yoga mat to the everyday details of our life.

Whether you want to lose weight and get fit, reduce stress and cope with life better, or explore your own spiritual path, yoga offers a way to cultivate personal awareness with more than physical relaxation. It is a pathway to a greater understanding of the question "Who am I?"

Comfortable clothing and a quiet place to practice are ideal. Yoga can be practiced anywhere at any time of the day or night. A morning practice is beneficial to prepare you for a new day filled with energy and focus. On the other hand, a practice in the evening helps to bring closure to the day. If you are a beginner or find that you need a little extra help to stretch your body, a strap and a sturdy blanket are good props to support you as you practice. The blanket can be folded into a cushion to sit on or can be used to cover you during Savasana. The strap will help you to reach those places where your stretch may not extend ... yet.

You can teach yourself the positions and breathing exercises in this book without an instructor, though I recommend that you seek out a teacher to help you learn some of the basics if you have never done yoga before. It is most helpful to have a "hands on" experience to help train your body to "feel" the poses.

It is not necessary to follow a guru or travel to India to practice yoga. It is as much about self-discovery as it is about learning from others. In yoga, the guru can be your practice itself. *Empowering Your Life with Yoga* gives you the simple tools and suggestions you need to begin a yoga practice or to enhance the practice you already have.

It is my wish that you will find endless sources of empowerment throughout your life.

"I honor you as I honor myself. I acknowledge we are all *One*."
—Namasté

How to Use This Book

The chapters in this book have been divided into two parts. The first part helps to explain what empowered living means through yoga, while the second part gives you a concrete guideline to follow, creating your own path to empowerment using the many tools of the yoga tradition.

You'll find the following elements in each chapter:

- A discussion of a particular yoga pose and how it relates to the contents of the chapter
- A simple yet profound empowerment exercise for you to try on your own, along with a discussion of the benefits and any cautions associated with each pose
- Inspiring real-life stories of aspiring yogis just like you
- Excerpts from the empowerment journals of my students or from my own experience
- Mantras for daily living—sacred sounds that are used to empower the mind and raise consciousness. Mantras can consist of a single syllable or a series of sounds and words, which may or may not have a meaning.

Although I have given detailed instructions for the yoga postures listed, I suggest that you use this book as a tool to enhance your personal yoga practice with an instructor to help give you physical direction and guidance. Follow your heart and feel the connection with your instructor.

This book can be used to support your yoga practice and to connect and empower you to your higher Self.

It is best to read this book from beginning to end to help put the concepts together more fluently; however, let the chapters guide you. If you feel particularly drawn to a certain chapter title, by all means, trust your intuition and start where you are!

Acknowledgments

I wish to thank Candy Paull for her most gracious and loving gift of friendship. Through her and this project, I have met new friends and colleagues who I am grateful for and whose talents and guidance have been invaluable.

Many thanks to Jacky Sach, my agent, for her trust in my abilities and for taking care of the "work" behind the scenes.

Mikal Belicove and Lynn Northrup, my editors, I am grateful for your patient guidance and encouragement.

To my beautiful family, friends, and fellow students scattered across this world, you continue to enrich me and I am blessed beyond measure.

Most of all, thank you Divine Spirit; through You, I am empowered!

Part One

What Is Empowered Living?

This book is organized into two main parts to give an overview of how yoga can empower your life. In addition, it shares a more detailed focus on some of the specific ways you can experience empowerment every day, on and off your yoga mat. Ultimately, though, you will feel empowerment long before you can analyze it, and this book can help you relate all the benefits of a yoga practice to the full potential in your life.

The chakras play an important role in empowering us to reach our highest potential through integration on many levels. In Chapter 1, we'll learn how these seven energy centers help to create and empower our life. In Chapter 2, we'll explore our dharma—the responsibility we take for our life. Chapter 3 will discuss how we accomplish our goals through our intentions and practices. This is our sadhana.

Come! Live the fully empowered life of yoga and see for yourself how rich life is!

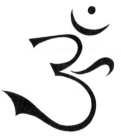

Chapter One

Focused Energy: Awakening to Possibility

What is our true nature? Our true nature is pure consciousness, the essence of our spirituality. Pure consciousness is an awareness we have that lies beyond thought, emotion, and the clutter that fills our everyday mind. By accessing this awareness we have the potential to achieve a spiritual focus we otherwise would not be capable of achieving.

Empowerment is the tool with which we reach this great potential and discover new possibilities. So how do we become empowered? We become empowered through self-knowledge. One of the most powerful ways of finding out who we are is through the body. Yoga, more than any physical exercise, can help us achieve this focused knowing.

Start Where You Are

At the height of laughter, the universe is flung into a kaleidoscope of new possibilities.

—Jean Houston, professor, scholar, and author

Taking a deep and soulful look at ourselves can be a difficult thing. As we peel away the layers of ego, judgment, fear, and self-consciousness, we are left with nothing but pure potential. It is frightening to let go of the conditioned thoughts we have accumulated over a lifetime: to release ourselves from the expectations of society, our parents, our community, and so on. These expectations become like a deeply grooved rut we get stuck in until one moment, one day, a spark of change ignites our thoughts and we are thrust outside of our own reality into a greater realm than what we had come to believe. Practices such as yoga, meditation, contemplation, and even stillness can be used to create an empowered life, to realize our full potential, and to awaken to all possibilities! The practice of yoga creates the focus we need to know ourselves at the deepest level of our true nature and release ourselves from the illusions we have carried about ourselves our entire lives.

Through movement, you engage your physical senses to "feel" life through your body, releasing old ideas to make room for new ones. Releasing means to surrender to what is. Releasing means acceptance of the here and now. That means, through your work with yoga, you accept the condition of your body, your life as it exists in the present moment, but you know that the ultimate goal is in achieving better health, more empowered relationships, and/or financial stability to bring your Spirit to wholeness. Instead of judging and clinging to our own righteousness and another's wrongs, we open our hands and hearts and let it all go. By releasing our obsessions with outer appearance, physical capabilities, and the images and judgments we have of ourselves, others, and our situations, we make room for a better self—our true Self—to emerge.

So where do we start? We start right here, in the now. We start where we are.

Less Is More

Sometimes less really is more. Letting go of striving and surrendering to the wisdom of your body will teach you lessons you'll never learn in books, lectures, and how-to courses. In yogic postures, your body becomes your teacher. Let go and let your body show you the way. In an asana (yoga pose), one part of the body is held strong, allowing another part to release, balancing between supporting and being supported. As you breathe into a pose and let go, you move more deeply into it. As you breathe deeply and relax into your life, you will discover the same lesson resonates within each situation you encounter. If you surrender to the situations that arise in your life, you will find yourself experiencing them in a deeper and more meaningful way.

Let your inner nature be the place where you rest. Cease doing and release into being. Stop striving and allow life to be exactly what it is right here, right now, in this moment. Pay attention to what is, not to regrets about what isn't or wishes about what could be. Empower yourself by being fully present and releasing all judgment and criticism. The energy of life will flow into the empty vessel, cleansing and renewing and releasing an inner power that does not depend on outer circumstances or self-limiting judgments.

Yoga helps your body release old tensions, memories of past trauma, and unconscious holding patterns such as old patterns of behavior that keep you from growing spiritually. This could be anything from nail biting to having an addiction of any kind. Breathing teaches you the open/close, inhale/exhale of tension and release. Each asana helps you to learn the art of releasing. For example, when you are depressed you tend to hunch forward and hang your head, hiding your heart, which creates even more tightness and depression. Standing in a yogic pose such as Tadasana (Mountain Pose, discussed later in this chapter) allows you to ground yourself, stand taller, expand your chest, and open your heart. As your body becomes more open, watch how grounded and compassionate you become toward the people in your life. Your relationship with your partner or your co-workers will develop a better sense of trust and kindness. In trusting your own foundation, you begin to relate better to others. What you do with your body reflects your attitude, and choosing to embody a different attitude will eventually make a difference in what you are thinking and feeling. Opening the body facilitates opening the mind and releasing energy that has gotten stuck. There is freedom in changing old attitudes—and that is empowering!

Making Way for the New

When you release the old, you make way for the new. Yoga moves you past your restrictive mental boxes into your body and eventually into your pure potential.

restrictive mental boxes
↓
pure potential

5

Whether you are a child exploring all the new adventures and opportunities of your world, a young adult beginning to realize your full potential, or a fully realized adult basking in the wisdom of your experience, it isn't too late to see how yoga can empower your life. You will never stop learning and experiencing new possibilities and opportunities until the day you transition from this world to the next, so there's no time like the present to get started. Wouldn't it be wonderful if you could move gracefully through life experiencing good health, fulfilling relationships, and a focus so precise that you are able to achieve your most treasured goals?

Now is the time to increase your focus, strengthen your concentration, and pay attention to your true nature. Yoga can help you achieve all three goals.

Practice: Focusing

The following are some steps you can take that will help you to focus your thoughts and intentions. As you keep your thoughts in one place for a period of time, you will find that things begin to happen in your life. Positive changes will occur and opportunities will present themselves to you.

1. Make a list of the five most treasured goals (or people) that you would like to have in your life.

2. Be as specific as you can with details, listing all the attributes you can think of that will bring these images into clear focus for you and will help you manifest your goals and intentions.

3. As you review your list, notice how you feel and in what part of your body the feeling is coming from. Are you content, joyful, at peace with, and/or happy with your intentions and desires? Do you feel empowered with your choices, or do you feel deprived because you do not have them yet? Where do you feel your feelings? Pay attention to your emotions and thoughts.

In taking a deeper look at your goals and intentions and how you react to them, you can see which ones are serving you and which ones are best to redefine. Actually focusing energy on your intentions will help you to surrender to the outcome.

Yoga is much more than physical postures and routines. It is traditionally referred to as a liberation teaching that seeks to release us from our limited view of Self. Yoga is a way of life that, in fact, does support good health, positive relationships, and personal achievement through concentrated and focused intention.

Directing Your Available Power

The word *focus*, according to *Webster's* dictionary, means "to concentrate" or "direct." Energy is defined as "available power." When we put these two words together, notice how empowering it is to "direct your available power" toward your intentions and goals. Yoga, meaning "union" or "integration," is exactly what we do when we "concentrate our available power." More than physical postures, yoga is a way of life in which we choose empowerment through our own choices, whether they are physical activities, emotional responses, or mental thoughts. Either way, yoga is an expression of our focused energy.

> ... and when we realize that our true Self is one of pure potentiality, we align with the power that manifests everything in the universe.
> —Deepak Chopra, best-selling author and physician

Chakras

Chakras are energy centers of the body that direct your available power into every aspect of your life. These little "wheels of light," as they are termed in the Sanskrit language, are vital to our health and well-being. They act as conductors, drawing vital energy from the earth, circulating it throughout the physical body, and then releasing it as our higher awareness. In other words, our chakras are the link in the process of receiving information, assimilating it, and applying it in a more refined sense. Their health and integrity are maintained through following a grounded lifestyle incorporating such physical exercises as yoga and being receptive to kind and loving thoughts and actions toward yourself and your surroundings.

The chakras are linked with the practice of yoga in that each yoga posture or breathing technique stimulates and/or soothes these energy centers. Let's explore yoga, the chakras, and how they interconnect to empower our lives on and off the mat.

What Are Chakras?

The word *chakra* signifies the place where mind and body meet and is based on the knowledge that all life is energy in varying degrees of density. Your chakras are constantly interacting with *all energy*, either inside of you or outside of you, to help keep your mind, body, and spirit healthy, focused, and receptive. These "wheels" are spinning energy centers located along the line of the spine, which affects many different levels of consciousness such as the emotional level, the mental level, and the physical level. They are a vital key to what we feel and think; however, they do not have a physical form. Since Western science has not yet been able to physically locate these "powerhouses" with their scopes, scans, and tests, the only proof you truly have of the existence of these energy centers are your own, direct experiences of energy in your life.

The practice of yoga stimulates these centers and the life themes they are associated with. For example, the first chakra relates to security. As you practice Tadasana, it stimulates the base of the spine and moves energy down your legs, which enforces feelings of being grounded. When you are physically grounded, you will feel secure with your place in life. You will feel supported in relationships from your job to your romantic interests and even your relationships with family and finances.

One of my students explained to me one day why he could not continue to come to yoga class. He was having a difficult time with his finances. Upon further discussion we uncovered that his financial instability stemmed from his perception of security. In his mind he felt he didn't have enough money to continue coming to class. He explained that he felt like a drifter and that his whole family had always suffered from an array of financial crises. He had convinced himself that his life would always be fraught with poverty.

I asked him to continue coming to class and offered that we concentrate on this area of his life and body. He accepted, and we immediately began working with his first chakra using yoga and pranayama as our foundation. Tadasana (Mountain Pose) and Virabadrasana (Warrior Pose, discussed in Chapter 5) were two of the main postures he worked with every day. We also incorporated a pranayama, Breath of Fire, also known as Kapalabhati Breath, to connect his body and mind and pull his power into himself. Breath of Fire engages the diaphragm as the practitioner forces breath through the nostrils by quickly pulling the abdomen inward. This creates a forceful breath which produces heat in the body.

Within one month's time, he began to see improvement not only in the strength and balance of his physical body, but he had found a better paying job and was beginning to save some money. This was nothing short of a miracle in his life and has empowered him to achieve more than he originally thought possible.

The chakras are located in the subtle body and relate closely with the nervous and endocrine systems, and have the ability to affect you through all elemental levels such as earth, water, fire, air, sound, light, and thought. The subtle body is not physically seen but surrounds the body. It is made up of energy that is less dense than our physical body.

The following table gives some basic information to help explain some of the functions and associations of the chakras.

Chakra Name	Theme	Element	Color
1st chakra—Root	Security	Earth	Red
2nd chakra—Sacral	Creativity/ Sexuality	Water	Orange
3rd chakra—Solar Plexus	Self-esteem	Fire	Yellow
4th chakra—Heart	Love	Air	Emerald green
5th chakra—Throat	Communication/ Self-expression	Sound	Sky blue
6th chakra—Third Eye	Intuition	Light	Indigo
7th chakra—Crown	Enlightenment	Thought	Violet

Picture the scene: A "busybody" co-worker has decided it is your turn to be the subject of the next office scandal. Your boss gets wind of the gossip and calls you into his office for a meeting. Your first reaction is to stand there dumbfounded, then your astonishment turns to anger at the false accusations but you can't let your boss see you lose your temper! What you'd rather do right now is run away screaming. You can feel an internal "shaking," and your legs turn to rubber (the threat of your security) and you have a lump in the pit of your stomach (fear of being disempowered). But you manage to take a few deep, full yogic breaths, pull yourself together, and calmly clear your name with your boss (and then face off with the co-worker). In doing so, you take on a strength and a calmness that empowers your spirit. This is an example of how your chakras can be affected through outside stimulation, and also how you can affect them with your internal responses and through your physical use of yoga (in this example, the deep breathing). Hopefully, however, rather than exercising the energy of our chakras through negative confrontation, we can start to transform the lower aspects of our nature into a higher, more loving and focused awareness.

Description of the Chakras

The following summary of each chakra will help you remember the areas of the body they affect, what they are associated with, and the related yoga postures used to balance them. There are seven chakras, beginning at the base of the spine and moving up to the crown of the head.

- The *first chakra* is located at the base of the spine (perineum) and relates to our security or foundation. Its related color is red and it is associated with the element of earth, which represents solidity, health, and survival. We have felt the effects of our first chakra when we have gone through periods of fear or loss. Changes of any kind can affect our first chakra because they "uproot" us and we lose that sense of groundedness. On the other hand, when our first chakra is powerful and balanced, we have a feeling that "all is right with the world" and that we have everything we need. As I mentioned earlier, Tadasana is an excellent posture to balance the first chakra and help you feel more secure. By standing tall and feeling the strength and suppleness of your spine, the body is reassuring your mind of a secure foundation.

- The *second chakra* is found in the lower abdomen (below the navel) and is associated with creativity, emotions, and sexuality. Its related color is orange and it corresponds with the element of water, which is associated with fluid bodily functions like circulation, elimination, and reproduction. Sometimes an overbearing sexual appetite or even a listless outlook on life can indicate an improperly functioning second chakra, but when you feel creative and joyful, that is when the second chakra is in balance. Pelvic rotations are excellent to balance the second chakra and to enhance your creativity. (Sit in a simple cross-legged position, placing your hands on your knees. As you inhale, lean forward and rotate to the right; exhale as you lean back and rotate to the left for as long as you feel comfortable. Repeat the sequence in the opposite direction, making sure to engage the stomach muscles.) When the pelvic region feels "stuck" or stiff, these rotations can move energy and release it through the sacral region. You will notice an increase in creativity and possibly a more balanced and healthy attitude regarding sexuality and your emotions.

The *third chakra* resides in the solar plexus and relates to our self-esteem and personal power. Its related color is yellow and the associated element is fire. In the body, fire relates to metabolism transforming matter into heat to create energy. Positive self-worth indicates a healthy third chakra, while low self-esteem is a strong indicator of improper functioning. Navasana (Boat Pose) and Setu Bandhasana (Bridge Pose) are excellent postures to support your solar plexus and foster a positive self-worth. Both postures directly affect your stomach through stretching and strengthening the power center.

To experience Navasana, sit with your legs extended in front of you, then bend your knees and draw them toward your chest, balancing on your sitbones. Place your hands under your knees as you begin to straighten your legs into the air and bring your body into a "V" shape. Be sure to tuck your navel toward your spine to support your lower back. To release, bend your knees and place the feet back on the floor.

Begin Setu Bandhasana by lying on your back with your knees bent and your feet as close to your buttocks as you can comfortably place them. Place your feet hip width apart and firmly press them into the floor as you lift your hips off the floor, slowly raising your spine from the tailbone upward to the shoulders. Press firmly into the feet and shoulders as you arch the belly and chest upward. Breathe deeply and hold for as long as is comfortable for you. Release by slowly lowering your spine back to the floor.

The *fourth chakra* is found in the sternum and is the place where we hold (unconditional) love. Emerald green is the fourth chakra's associated color and air is the related element. Our breath is closely related to air; it is the life-giving force that sustains all functions of the body. Grief and sadness along with stooped shoulders are important indications of an improperly functioning fourth chakra, while the feelings of joy, compassion, and unconditional love show its healthy functioning. Ustrasana (Camel Pose, discussed in Chapter 4) is one of the most powerful poses to balance the fourth chakra and to open yourself to love because of the intense stretch it gives across your chest.

- The *fifth chakra*, located in the throat, is associated with communication and self-expression. Its related color is sky blue and the associated element is sound. Sound is created through vibration, which every being can feel. This is our most elemental form of communication. Think about those times when you found yourself tongue-tied when you wanted to say something really important and couldn't. Those were the times when your fifth chakra was not vibrating at its full potential. Likewise, when your throat is clear of frogs and you can easily articulate what you want to say, you can be assured that your fifth chakra is strong. Ustrasana (Camel Pose) is also good to balance the fifth chakra as you drop your head back and stretch through and stimulate the throat.

- The *sixth chakra* is found in the center of the forehead (an area that's known as the "third eye") and is linked to intuition and imagination. This chakra is related to the color indigo and is associated with the element of light. Light is a much more refined vibration and relates to our intuition. When you trust your intuition and act on your hunches, you are using your sixth chakra energy, but when you second-guess yourself or get stuck in outdated modes of thinking, the sixth chakra is not functioning properly. Yoga mudra (discussed in Chapter 2) can help balance your sixth energy center by focusing your awareness between your eyes as you bow forward.

- The *seventh chakra* is located at the top of the head and relates to knowledge and transcendent consciousness. It is associated with the color violet and the element of thought. Thought, or consciousness, relates to our ability to reason and to move beyond the limitations of the mind and into Spirit. That expansive feeling of being connected to everything is a powerful indication that your seventh chakra is supporting you; however, when you feel separated from your spirit and life seems to lose meaning for you, your seventh chakra may be closed. Savasana (Corpse Pose, discussed in Chapter 11) can help you to reconnect and balance the seventh energy center. When you surrender in Savasana and breathe with Ujjayi Breath, you release the mind from all the internal chatter and allow yourself to rest in complete awareness of all that is.

Chakra-Balancing Exercise

Our best preparation for tomorrow is the proper use of today.
—Anonymous

This exercise can be done before you begin your yoga practice to help deepen the effects of the physical postures. By setting the intentions for each chakra and the corresponding bodily areas, you are creating a synergistic connection between mind, body, and emotions. Take your time through this exercise and notice the subtle changes that occur within you on all levels.

Sit or recline comfortably with your spine straight, eyes closed, and begin to take some deep breaths to clear out your lungs and to focus your awareness into your body. As your thoughts release and you are focused only on your breath, turn your awareness to the base of your spine and focus there for a few breaths, visualizing the color red. As you begin to feel your tailbone relax, take one or two more breaths and set your intention for the first chakra: *Security.*

Now, move your awareness to your lower abdomen, just below the navel, and focus your breathing into that area as you visualize the color orange. Notice the sensations in this area. As you feel yourself relax, continue breathing and set your intention for the second chakra: *Creativity.*

Gently shift your awareness to your solar plexus and focus your breathing. Feel your belly rise and fall with each full breath and as you do, visualize the color yellow. As with the previous chakras, notice the sensations here and notice as your abdomen relaxes. Your belly may start to feel warm. Set your intention for the third chakra: *Self-esteem.*

Continue your deep breathing as you move your focus to your sternum. Notice how your chest rises and falls as you breathe. Visualize the color emerald green and focus on the feelings of your chest, heart, and lungs. When relaxation washes over you, set your intention with the words: *Unconditional love.*

Bring your awareness to your throat and feel your breath flowing through your windpipe. As you feel it move through you, visualize the color sky blue and feel as if your throat is expanding into relaxation. Feel your breath flowing more freely and make your intention: *Self-expression*.

With your eyes still closed, turn your inner gaze to your forehead and continue breathing, focusing your breaths on the spot between your eyes. Visualize the color indigo blue and feel the sensations of release and relaxation melt across your forehead. Make your intention with the word: *Intuition*.

Finally, place your inner gaze at the top of your head and feel your breath flowing in and out from that point. In your mind's eye, see the color violet at the crown of your head. As your head relaxes, make your intention with the word: *Enlightenment*.

Continue breathing deeply and let all the colors you have visualized melt into a brilliant, white light. See yourself breathe in the white light and feel it permeate every cell of your body. Let yourself rest in that image until you feel ready to open your eyes. Slowly open your eyes and stretch your body in ways it's asking you to move. Notice that you feel calmer and more balanced.

This exercise can be done anywhere to help bring you back to a place of calm center. Many comments from my students suggest that this visualization technique has made the difference for them between a hectic, unempowered day versus having a more focused, loving outlook on life. I use this visualization at the end of many yoga classes while the students are in Savasana to enforce a deeper transformational experience. Go ahead, give it a try!

A View from the Mountain Top

Can you think of a time in your life when you felt so good that you could hardly believe your experiences? Picture the first time you landed a job you really wanted, or when you graduated from college or got married, and remember how you felt. Didn't it give you a sense of empowerment? Do you remember that quiet, grounded yet reverent feeling of being totally alive? Yes!

I remember how I felt the first time I hiked to the top of a 14,000-foot mountain in Colorado. Full of strength and feeling "one" with the mountain, I stood there in awe at the expansiveness around me and of the energy inside me. It was a magnificent experience that every cell of my body recorded and can now recall whenever I remember that magical time.

By the same token, yoga activates all aspects of you in ways that energize, heal, and empower you to live fully and with grace. As a matter of fact, I'd be willing to bet that you do yoga every day without realizing what it is you are doing.

I am beginning to learn that it is the sweet, simple things of life which are the real ones after all.
—Laura Ingalls Wilder, author

Take the simple act of standing, for instance. Do a quick body scan and see if you're standing equally on both feet with your tummy tucked in. Notice if your chest is expanded and your shoulders are relaxed down your back. Is your head lifted or are you looking downward? These are all positions of Tadasana, Mountain Pose. Remember how you felt on top of that peak? You can recreate that feeling just by adjusting your standing posture to reflect the strength and majesty of the mountain.

Tadasana (Mountain Pose)

Tadasana helps to create stability and supports the first chakra. Notice how your mind becomes calmer and your emotions even out when you are standing tall with a straight spine. An erect spine allows energy to flow through you in an uninterrupted path. That means you are better able to receive and let the energy of health, creativity, focused thought, and centered calm flow through you. It also opens up the chakra connection in your body. Each chakra vibrates, emanating energy through the spine and to all parts of you, from your internal organs to your mental thoughts and even expanding to your emotions.

Tadasana makes you a better energy conductor. Liken it to a power line. Electricity flows through the straight power lines but it will flounder and short out when the line is broken or knotted up. Imagine how that misguided energy could hurt someone! It is the same way with the energy in your body. When you stand erect and breathe deeply, you are allowing energy to flow freely through your body. But when you slouch your shoulders, reach your head forward, or even stand on one leg, you create places in your body where the energy gets stuck, thus creating stiff joints and muscles, or worse yet, weakened chakras that have trouble supporting all the systems of your body. When the body is stiff, so are the emotions and the mind, and when you are experiencing your life from restriction, notice how events and situations arise in your life that cause blockages.

On the other hand, when you relax your body through yoga, such things as better health, an open heart to your loved ones, or greater understanding in your chemistry class become easier to accomplish.

Being a Mountain

Tadasana brings stamina, focus, balance, groundedness, and patience to your life. Use it when you get up in the mornings to prepare yourself to face the challenge of a new day. Let it balance you physically so you can "feel" your body before you set off on your daily adventures. Let it focus you mentally, bringing your thoughts into the present moment so you can make clear, honest, and understandable decisions. Let it ground you emotionally in those times when fear threatens to throw you off course in your personal relationships, your career, or even with your physical health. Also, let Tadasana give you patience for those times when you are dealing with such situations as the tantrums of your two-year-old or the rush-hour traffic on your way home from work.

When you change your consciousness, you change the way you approach everything from diet and exercise to health, career, and love. The positive possibilities are endless in your life when you become centered, focused, and aware in body, mind, and spirit. Yoga is a total workout for your entire being. Let it empower your life with the limitless possibilities you were born to live!

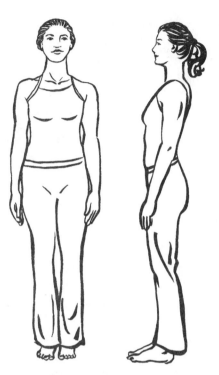

Tadasana (Mountain Pose).

Empowerment Exercise: Tadasana

Tadasana Affirmation: *I am balanced in body, mind, and spirit, which roots me into the earth and releases me to all possibilities!*

Tadasana may look like an easy pose that doesn't have many benefits, but if you practice it with mindfulness and pay attention to all the sensations of your body as you adjust and relax into the posture, you will find there is great strength and energy in this pose.

1. To come into this asana, stand up straight with your <u>feet together</u>. Make sure your toes are pointing forward and your feet are parallel.

2. Slightly turn your <u>thighs inward</u> as you <u>tuck</u> your tailbone. This will ground your weight more fully into your legs and will strengthen your lower abdominal muscles.

3. Without sticking out your belly, lift your chest and pull your shoulders back, feeling as if the bottom tips of your shoulders are moving toward each other. (Keep breathing!)
4. Keep your chin parallel to the floor and draw your head back over your shoulders.
5. Take a deep breath in and as you exhale, soften your buttocks. Make sure your gaze is focused yet soft.
6. Stand in Tadasana for approximately 5–8 rounds of breath or as long as you desire.

Benefits

Some of the benefits you will experience as you practice Tadasana will be subtle, while others will have an almost immediate, profound effect. With practice, it improves your balance and posture, promoting deeper breathing, which will in turn relax and calm the mind. As you continue the practice of Tadasana, you will notice greater leg strength and improved physical balance as well as a greater mental balance. In turn, your life seems to take on an "ease." Household chores are accomplished with greater ease, work becomes interesting, and it is a joy to spend time with your loved ones. And, oh yes, you will find that you have more time to just "be" than you ever thought you had. Through energetic focus, you've organized your life so that you actually fit into the picture!

I usually practice this pose when my focus is harder to hold on to and I need to get grounded. This is excellent to do anywhere, whether you are standing in line at the grocery store, painting in your art class, or at work. With only a few breaths and the correct posture, you will find that your body releases the stress it had been holding and your mind quickly comes back to focus.

Cautions

If you're pregnant, overweight, or have an injury or diagnosed illness, please check with your doctor before beginning your yoga practice.

There aren't too many cautions where Tadasana is concerned; however, be careful not to lock or hyperextend the knees. It is possible that you could pass out if you kept your knees locked for a long period of time.

Instead, allow a slight, comfortable release in this area and this pose will energize as well as give you roots for an active, standing posture.

Life is what we make it, always has been, always will be.
—Grandma Moses, U.S. painter

Real Life

This example comes from my experience one Christmas Eve afternoon a few years ago. The stress levels were high throughout the entire facility!

"I was standing in line at the airport in Nashville, Tennessee, on a busy, snowy holiday weekend. The line was snaking through the terminal and had started to extend outside! I found myself in the middle of this line with barely enough time to catch my flight. My breathing had gotten shallow and I was clenching my teeth *and* my rear end! My holiday spirits had begun to droop as I felt my temper rise for fear that I would miss my flight. As I shifted from one foot to the other, "BINGO!" I realized how I was standing and could feel, all of a sudden, how tight and stressed my body was feeling! I immediately stood on both my feet, tucked my tummy and tailbone, lifted my chest and took a *huge* breath in as slow and as full as I could make it. As I began to exhale, my shoulders began to relax and drop down my back. My facial muscles began to soften and so did my anger. A couple more breaths and I almost had forgotten about the long line ahead of me. A few more breaths and my mind began to focus on a solution to my problem rather than the problem itself. Within minutes I regained my composure, felt more confident and compassionate, and I walked up to the ticket counter, apologized to the agent and the next person in line for butting in and explained my situation. As the agent looked up, her irritated look softened because I approached her in a composed and compassionate way. Even the next person in line felt compassion for me and ushered me ahead! As it turned out, I made my flight with 10 minutes to spare!

I was able to turn a very challenging situation into something I could work with, just by changing my breathing patterns and the way I held my body. The physical change in turn triggered the relaxation response in my brain, which allowed me to stay focused and calm and achieve my goal!"

Empowerment Journal

An important tool to help you track your progress to empowerment throughout the day/week/month is a journal in which you can note all the times you felt empowered during your yoga workout. This can be anything from a simple, spiral-bound notebook to a more decorative journal found in a bookstore. You can even keep a journal on your computer, if you prefer. Use your journal to make lists of your physical feelings, thoughts, emotions, where the feelings are located, and what triggered certain situations to stand out as you held a particular pose. In this chapter we will concentrate more closely on Tadasana.

> Every breath we take, every step we make, can be filled with peace, joy and serenity. We need only be awake, alive in the present moment.
> —Thich Nhat Hanh, Vietnamese Buddhist monk and author

Recording these experiences in a journal ultimately gives you clues to the progress you are making in your life. For instance, let's say you felt particularly wobbly while standing in Tadasana today. How did it make you feel? Write down the places in your body where you noticed sensations. Did you have a tightness in your hips or did your legs feel weak? Once you jot down your thoughts and feelings from this pose, apply the aspects of the first chakra to your experience to see how and where you are being affected. Feeling weak in the knees could show that you don't feel very secure with some aspect of your home, family, finances, or love life, and it may tell you something about how you relate to change. On the other hand, if your Mountain Pose was solid and you felt stable and strong, you can be pretty sure that your first chakra is balanced and there is harmony in areas of your home, family, and career.

Don't judge yourself or your reactions, but just notice and become aware of how you react. You are the observer in your own life and therefore can see the areas that might need a little more attention.

Here is an excerpt from Pam's empowerment journal for you to use as an example to get you started with your journal. She has been a student of mine for nearly three years and I am encouraged by her dedication to her practice and how it has affected her life:

There I stood, thinking that finally my teacher calls for Mountain Pose. At last, we are able to simply stand. As I am looking forward to this lazy Mountain Pose, I have a lightning strike revelation! I realize that Mountain Pose is very active. Spiraling thighs, tucked pelvic girdle, relaxed shoulders and neck, tucked chin ... balance, balance. I look forward to this pose at first because it is a chance to rest, however I realize that I look for this pose because it integrates all of what yoga means to me .... Gentle, solid work, with calmness and strength.

Using this pose in day to day life has become a retreat to calmness and peace. I am able to find my Mountain Pose in those few moments when I am still in my busy life. I even find it when I begin to lose my temper or am looking for my patience! Mountain Pose is a simple retreat into a strong, calm, peaceful place for which I am grateful.

Mantras for Daily Living

A mantra is a sacred sound, word, phrase, or chant that resonates with the spirit. It serves as a focusing device for calming the mind and is designed to awaken the mind from its habitual unconsciousness. It helps to raise your energy vibrations to support transformational experiences, whether they are minor or life changing. Mantras directly affect the vibrations of the chakras by balancing their energy. Sound waves can and do affect matter, so it's not surprising that they would affect your consciousness as well.

The essence of all beings is earth, the essence of earth is water, the essence of water is plants, the essence of plants is man, the essence of man is speech, the essence of speech is the Holy Knowledge (Veda) the essence of Veda is Sama-Veda (word, tone, sound), the essence of Sama-Veda is OM.
—*Chandogya Upanishad*, ancient yogic text

It is not necessary to intellectualize the meaning of a mantra for the sound to have an effect on you. The rhythms of the sound work subconsciously to break old patterns and create new ways of thinking and being. Part of the magic of a mantra is in not thinking about its meaning, but allowing the sound to reverberate through you, trusting that on a sub-conscious level you are coming to a place of healing and balance. If, how-ever, you choose a mantra that has meaning for you, such as "I am peace," the rhythm of the repetition will help to infuse its meaning into your consciousness.

Once you choose the mantra(s) that you feel compelled to use, try re-peating it (focusing on one mantra at a time, if you're using more than one) out loud. Spoken aloud for a few minutes in the morning can move silently through your mind all day, carrying with it the imprints of its vibration, image, and meaning. You can even recite your mantra while practicing yoga, and then continue the mantra as you go through your day, which will deeply instill the benefits of your physical practice. The act of chanting itself instills the intention of your mantra into all aspects of your consciousness.

Here are some examples of mantras you may want to use to empower yourself as you move through the situations of your life. These particular selections relate to the different chakras. Don't feel limited to this list. Feel free, even empowered, to make up your own mantra(s) as you see fit.

- "OM, Shanti, Shanti." ("All of existence is peace, peace.")
- "SAT NAM." ("I am truth.")
- "I accept myself as I am."
- "I allow abundance into my life."
- "I use my power wisely."
- "Love underlies all possibilities."
- "I speak only my truth."
- "I trust my intuition."
- "I acknowledge the presence of Spirit working through me."
- "I am balanced in my being which releases me to all possibilities."
- "Through patience, I can achieve all my goals."

You may be wondering, "What if I don't have a good voice?" It doesn't matter whether or not you sound like an opera singer. It doesn't even mat-ter if you can't carry a tune in a bucket. What does make a difference in your mantra recitation is the fact that you do it with intention and rever-ence. Take about five minutes and repeat your mantra as you practice your favorite yoga pose. Then notice how the rest of your day unfolds. You just might be surprised to find your true voice!

The Possibilities Are Endless

Do you find yourself taking the same route to work every day? Maybe you have fallen into a routine that shuts off your senses and makes you feel like one day is pretty much the same as all the rest. If you have a structured routine, change it around every once in a while to move you out of complacency and into new, innovative thoughts. Do you believe that miracles are a thing of the past? Do you live for your two-week vacation once a year? If you can say "yes" to these questions, it may be time to wipe the sleep out of your eyes and wake up to the endless possibilities that are available to you through conscious and focused choice.

In the words of the late sage and founder of Integral Yoga, Swami Satchidananda: "Paths are many—Truth is ONE." Let your life be one in which you find Truth through many different avenues of possibility. Yoga is one way in which you can open yourself up to all possibilities through the experiences of not only your physical body, but of your mental and emotional bodies as well.

Prepare different foods, try different restaurants, take a class that you're interested in just because you want to learn more. Practice a new yoga posture that you have been too afraid to try ... until now! Try to see particular situations in different ways, expect the unexpected, and don't assume anything! You just might surprise yourself with all the new creativity and wisdom that you uncover.

Yoga does not simply reveal the possibilities of our potential. It actually activates the potential hidden deep within, thus enhancing the range of possibilities that are available to us. Yoga empowers us to live a deeper, richer, more satisfying life, merely by waking up to what we already hold within us.

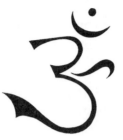

Chapter Two

Discipline: Intention Is Everything

Intention is an attitude and literally affects how we interpret what comes into our mind. Setting our intention is based on what matters most to us. It is made by a commitment to align our thoughts and actions with our values. When setting intentions we must live them every day. They are like muscle—we build it over time with use, but if we neglect it, it becomes weak and we must start over again. Likewise, our intentions become weak and less focused when we do not follow thought with deed.

align thoughts with values

It is important for us to know the difference between intention and goal-setting. Although goals are valuable and help us to apply discipline to attain future outcomes, intention is a practice that is focused in the "now" and reflects our state of being. For example, your goal may be to perform a headstand with precision in the middle of a room, while your intention is placed on your breath and your alignment as you attempt the posture in the moment.

The soul's ultimate intention is its expression of the true Self. In that expression we discover that by living our intentions in the present moment, we find our purpose in life. This purpose is called dharma.

Dharma

Dharma is a Sanskrit term meaning "purpose in life." It is also associated to the teachings of Buddhism and refers to the impermanent and inter-dependent nature of all life. Our everyday experiences bring these teachings to reality through the constantly changing events of our lives. Living your dharma is about the compassion that naturally arises when you reflect deeply on what it means to be alive. That means, as we reflect on and accept the good times of our life, we also look at and accept the challenges too. Yoga can assist us in our journey of impermanence by strengthening our physical body and increasing our overall health so that we may live fully and approach our challenges with understanding and resolve. Through yoga we calm the emotions, clear the scattered thoughts of the mind, and fortify the body for this human experience. Our spirits have chosen the physical experience of being human to fulfill a specific purpose on earth, and with that comes the knowledge that nothing stays the same.

> You are what your deep, driving desire is.
> As your desire is so is your will.
> As your will is, so is your deed.
> As your deed is, so is your destiny.
> —*Brihadaranyaka Upanishad*, ancient yogic text

There are three aspects to dharma. The first aspect says that each of us is here to discover our true Self. The second aspect of dharma is to express our individual talents, and the third aspect is being of service to humanity. Through practicing yoga we come to know our bodies, minds, and emotions more intimately, allowing for us to make better decisions about our paths. When we approach our life in this manner—discovering, expressing, and being of service—we experience empowerment, which is the ultimate goal of our Spirit. Through empowerment we can know the ecstasy of "being."

You may be thinking, this is all good, but how do I know my true Self and what are my talents? The tools in this book give you some very good ways to help you understand yourself better and to actually figure out what it is that really empowers you. Yoga is one of the main ingredients to help bring to light the questions you may have of following your dharma.

Through the practice of yoga, not only will you experience changes in your body, but you will begin to notice the subtle workings of your mind and your emotions. Thoughts will become clearer, concepts will open up to you like they never have before, and your emotional well-being will be more stable and you can act from a place of centeredness instead of an emotional whirlwind.

I remember when I took my first yoga class. I was in college and had to have a physical education credit to graduate. Since I wasn't into team sports like baseball and volleyball, that didn't leave much for me to choose from. Tennis was an option, but then I came across a beginning yoga class that fit perfectly with my schedule so I signed up, not really knowing what to expect.

What followed was nothing short of a total life-changing experience! From the first class I ever took, the change in me was immediate and profound. I walked away from that first class feeling more alive and focused than I had ever felt before. I had never even realized that one body could stretch and relax so deeply in an hour and a half. Until you experience yoga for yourself it may sound like an exaggeration, but there was no denying for me that I had found something that my Spirit had been searching for without even realizing it, and my body was also reaping the benefits of flexibility, strength, and tone.

As I continued my dedicated practice, other more subtle changes began to occur, until one day I realized that the motivations for my life were changing and I no longer simply existed in my life, I was fully "living" it. My grades improved and my job seemed more fun. Even my eating habits changed without any forcing. I found that I naturally gravitated toward lighter, more "alive" foods. I could actually taste the difference between "dead" food such as meats and processed food compared to fruits, vegetables, and whole grains that gave me more energy. I even noticed that my circle of friends was changing effortlessly. People who I no longer had much in common with just seemed to move in a different direction from me, while people who shared more of my values just "showed up"!

In becoming more aware of how I was living my life, I began to contemplate "who I am" and "why I am here." Through those contemplations I not only came to know my Self, but I began to realize those things in life that gave me great joy—my talents and gifts. It is through those talents that I have discovered what I share with humanity and thus profess my dharma—my purpose in life.

Let's take a deeper look into our true Selves and feel the empowerment as we discover who we are, express our gifts, and share them with others.

Discovering Your True Self

Part of our dharma is to find out that our true Self is spiritual. Essentially, we are spiritual beings that have taken on physical form in order to realize very important aspects of ourselves. We are not human beings having intermittent spiritual experiences. We are, in fact, spiritual beings having occasional human experiences. We are learning through our physical expressions, such as yoga, meditation, and loving kindness, that inside of us is a spark that wants to be born so that we can express our divinity.

It is right and necessary that we should be individuals. The Divine Spirit never made any two things alike—no two rosebushes, no two snowflakes, two grains of sand or two persons. We are all just a little unique for each wears a different face; but behind each is the One Presence—God.
—Ernest Holmes, author

Haven't you noticed that after you walk out of a yoga class you smile more? Or perhaps you have forgotten about that altercation you had with the parking attendant and realize that it just doesn't matter anymore. The change to your daily life might even be so subtle that you don't notice any big difference in what is happening to you, but what is different is the way you look at life. Whether or not you can finally do a headstand or touch your hands to your toes is not the main emphasis, but it is the process with which we find our dharma and create peace in our lives. The teachings of yoga explain that if your life as a whole has become easier, happier, and/or more focused, then your practice on the mat is working.

Following dharma also tells us not to hide from the challenges in our lives. By meeting them head-on and honestly looking at them, we come to know ourselves through our own right action. An example of meeting a challenge head on while practicing on the mat might be that you are working with tight hamstrings and find that forward bending is difficult for you. It may be difficult for you to fold into Uttanasana (Standing

Forward Bend) without having to bend your knees. Your lower back muscles may feel tight and your hamstrings feel more like rocks than rubber bands. This can make you anxious and want to judge yourself for not being as flexible as you want to be. However, as you physically and mentally stay with this posture, breathing in and relaxing into it on each exhale, you begin to notice the subtle shifts occurring in your hips and legs. Each breath allows your body to release more into the pose. You are actually feeling progress happening with each breath no matter how small the movement.

Now, let's apply the work you just accomplished with your hamstrings to your daily life. The fact that you worked through the challenge of tight hamstrings without giving up not only creates stamina, determination, and patience on the mat, it filters into your personal and professional life as well. Notice how you have more patience with your children or with your spouse after a long day on the job. Notice how empowered you feel as you create and follow through with projects at work with more determination and the stamina to see them through to completion. Become aware of the greater stamina you have throughout your day. You might no longer feel exhausted after lunch and need to take naps.

It is not what happens to us in life, but what we choose to do about it that reveals our true Self. The same is true in the practice of yoga. As you breathe into and stretch to your limits in any given pose, you will find the confidence and grace to flow through your challenges on the mat, as well as in your daily life, turning them into wisdom.

Think of a major challenge that you have recently gone through and ask yourself how well you approached the problem. Maybe you just went through a breakup, or lost your job, or can't see eye-to-eye with your best friend or partner. Either way, recall a situation without judging yourself for your actions, but merely take note of your reaction to the situation. Did you keep a calm head or did you lose your temper? Were you trusting that "everything would be all right" or did you immediately jump to the conclusion that "all was lost"?

The answers to these questions can help to give you insight into yourself. By taking the time to practice Ujjayi Breath (Ocean Breath) or a centering pose like Vrkasana (Tree Pose), you will be able to see the areas of your life that are in the process of being transformed and you will also see glimpses of your true Self. By collecting information from those times when you approached life with trust, calmness, and patience (to name a few) on and off the mat, you come to know who you really are and can then explore the many gifts and talents that are already inherent in your being.

Expressing Your Unique Talents

Everyone has a purpose in life, a special talent or gift that they alone can share with the world. No one is exempt from having a special gift; however, many of us have not truly found our special talent. According to dharma, you have a unique way of expressing the talent(s) you have. There is something that you can do better than anyone else in the world and it is important that you fulfill your purpose.

> The Divine Spirit is flowing through me in an individual way and I accept the genius of my own being.
> —Ernest Holmes, author

So how do you come to realize your talents? You find your talents through an understanding of yourself. Yoga is the perfect step in helping you realize what you have to offer the world. To begin with, the simple act of breathing takes your focus from outside of yourself and brings it into your body, connecting it with your mind and emotions. We've all heard the line "take a deep breath" when we were trying to calm down from some uncomfortable situation. There is merit to that statement, and it is the main component in the practice of yoga.

Once you can focus on your inner feelings and thoughts because of your breathing techniques, you then can use the movement of yoga to explore your abilities. For example, think of a time when you practiced a particularly difficult balancing posture and you kept falling out of the pose but kept working with it until your form was clean and your mind was focused. Through your mat practice you developed stamina and came to realize that you have determination and focus to follow through with a posture. Apply that to your daily life now and see the wonderful talent you have by seeing a project through to the finish at work. This makes you a reliable and dependable employee with leadership qualities that any boss would want to have on staff.

When you express your unique gift(s), it takes you into the realm of timelessness. Everything you do in the name of your life's purpose will seem natural to you and will flow from you like water from an open dam.

Think about the activities you do in a single day and reflect on what actually gives you joy and empowerment. Unique talents come in all shapes and sizes and relate to anything in life, from having the ability to crunch numbers and relate to economics to being intuitive with animals and children, and everything in between.

As you can see, talent is vast and comes in many different forms. Take the time to find and nurture what talents lie inside of you and then bring them out to express the fullness of who you are. A yoga practice can be an excellent way for you to uncover and even enhance your gifts. Think about the yoga poses that you are drawn to. Do you find yourself standing in headstand or handstand often because you like the way it feels to be upside down? Maybe these inversions are empowering you to look at life from a different point of view. Notice how innovative and open-minded you are with projects at work or even with your own artistic talents. The process of yoga is meant to bring about a profound transformation through the transcendence of your ego. *transcendence of ego*

Dedicating Yourself to Serving Others

The third aspect of dharma is service to humanity—to do for others and to ask yourself the questions, "How may I serve?" or "How can I help?" When you combine your talent with your willingness to serve, you are making a choice, and this is the very heart of service. You are making full use of your dharma.

> Therefore always perform unattached the deed to be done. For the man who performs action without attachment obtains the Supreme.
> —The *Bhagavad-Gita*, 3:19

We've all heard the saying "Do what you love and the money will follow." There is a deep element of truth to this statement, for it shows that if we live our lives through the expressions of our talents and gifts, serving others as we are able, then we will enjoy abundance in all areas of our lives. It is especially apparent in the connection we share with our work.

However, this does not mean that we are motivated strictly by the benefits we could receive from our actions, but we act because we have someone else's best interests at heart.

Let's put a different little twist to this service to humanity. As you come to your mat, ask your yoga practice "How may I serve?" and dedicate your service to the highest potential of your yoga workout. When you approach your practice with such dedication and focus, notice how you feel at the end of class. Then see if it filters into your daily life either with more compassion toward your co-workers, friends, and family, or even having more kindness and compassion toward yourself.

It is dedicating our talents to the service of others that brings us to the realization that we are all connected. We are all *One*.

The Art of Discipline

Discipline has less to do with accomplishment and more to do with intention and commitment. In other words, it matters more in your yoga practice if you make a commitment to show up to the mat on a daily basis with the intention of experiencing rather than accomplishing. Yoga can be achieved through practice and detachment in that practice. As it is with your daily life, your peace of mind and happiness are short-lived if all you are concerned about is the quantity of your accomplishments. Is it not "a job well done" with the intention of service and right action that truly gives you peace? Doesn't it matter more that you actually attempted your yoga practice instead of perfecting a handstand?

> We need a repeated discipline, a genuine training, in order to let go of our old habits of mind and to find and sustain a new way of seeing.
> —Jack Kornfield, author

All of life is practice, and your practice is discipline in action. It is not about what you get, but what you give. It is expressed by the intention to stay present in each moment. Whether it is waking up at 6:00 A.M. to get your children off to school, making sure that your house is clean for company, making time for your meditation practice, or paying bills, you are practicing intention. Likewise, practicing yoga in a class or on your own, or taking 10 minutes to do nothing but focus on your breathing, done with deep intimacy in each moment, leads you to discipline.

Without intimacy, you are merely acting like a robot. It has been said that laziness is not a matter of doing nothing, but is being so busy that you do not have time to smile at a stranger. Discipline, then, is quality of action, not quantity of work. It is doing what is possible with consistency. If you do what you can in your life (and on the mat) and do it fully, you will experience a sense of transformation and freedom, which is the reason for all discipline.

Making Commitments to Yourself

How many times have you put someone else's needs before your own only to feel hurt or resentment because your needs weren't met? It's true that through some of our commitments, like raising our children, we must consider most of their needs first. However, think of those times when your neighbor just dropped over unannounced and asked if you would donate to this cause or volunteer for that function and you said yes out of guilt or unrealistic obligation. Or how about the time you were on your way out the door to your yoga class when a friend called to tell you all about her terrible boss and you missed class because you couldn't figure out a good way to get her off the phone? (I feel you cringing right now!) Don't judge yourself, we've all done this a time or two in our lives. First of all, we broke the commitment of speaking our truth and then, as we felt resentful for being pushed into the situation, we broke the commitment to ourselves by not taking responsibility for our own choices.

> The primary method to overcome social afflictions is self-discipline in personal life, through which one attempts to master self-control; it is very difficult to impose discipline from the outside.
> —His Holiness the 14th Dalai Lama, Tenzin Gyatso

The next time you feel that you are not honoring the commitments you made to yourself, take a look at your yoga practice. Are you still going to class regularly or have you been skipping class here and there because of "other obligations"? Are you putting your full attention into each posture that you move into, or is your mind wandering to other things while you press into a Downward Dog?

You can bet your yoga practice and your life will mirror each other. Once you make a commitment to put your full attention in your practice, it will be much easier to make the commitment to yourself in your life.

The lessons here are simple. Keep your word with yourself. Take responsibility for your own choices instead of waiting for someone else to make things happen. Have the belief that you are just as valuable as anyone else and you do not have to do what someone else says if it doesn't feel right to you. These are attitudes that say "I am living in my power and I honor myself as I honor my neighbor."

Making Commitments to Others

I like to practice partner yoga to help me evaluate and keep my commitments to others. Don't let the term "partner yoga" confuse you. You don't have to have a spouse or life partner to practice partner yoga. It's not about sex and intimate romantic relationships (Tantra Yoga covers those subjects), but it does concentrate on relating and committing.

> The need for devotion to something outside ourselves is even more profound than the need for companionship ... we all must have some purpose in life; for no man can live for himself alone.
> —Ross Parmenter, American music critic and writer

When you engage in the practice of partner yoga, you are in a sense surrendering your own separate will for that of the partnership. You are "showing up" for the good of the whole and you become aware of the other person's weaknesses and strengths, as he or she becomes aware of yours.

As you practice the Tree Pose together, for example, both partners are relying on the stability of the other partner for their balance. Without the joined effort, the commitment to support each other, the pose would fall apart and your tree would topple to the ground. With commitment, both partners trust in their own abilities and in those of the other. Continued partner yoga practice will give you the empowered feeling of stepping up to the plate and honoring your commitments whether they are on the mat or in your daily life.

Practice: Commitment ✪

In your journal, make a list of the people and causes you are committed to, whether it's your spouse, children, a friend, colleagues, job, or a special interest group. Ask yourself if the commitments you made to these people and organizations honor you. If you feel any resentment at all toward anything, it's time to take a look at and re-evaluate your commitments.

> Until one is committed, there is hesitancy ... the moment one definitely commits oneself, then Providence moves too. All sorts of things occur to help one that would never otherwise have occurred.
>
> —Johann Wolfgang von Goethe, German poet, dramatist, and novelist

Resentment has no place in a commitment and is a major reason for humanity's feelings of separateness. When you feel any negativity with regard to a promise that you've made, locate that feeling in your body. Once you find it, breathe into it and stretch that area to release the negative feeling. I'll use the example of Ardha Matsyendrasana (Half Spinal Twist) to explain my point. (This pose will be discussed in detail in Chapter 3.)

Say, for instance, as you were evaluating your commitment to your job your belly started aching on the right side (your liver area). Then you realized you were feeling angry and resentful toward a co-worker who had been taking too much time off work, which left you with your job *and* hers to do. Since you did not honor the boundary of your promise to yourself and overextended your commitment to someone who did not appreciate you, no wonder you don't feel good about your choices!

Now is the time to start making amends to yourself and sit down on your yoga mat and breathe. The flushing sensation of Ardha Matsyendrasana will stimulate and stretch the area of your liver to help release some of that anger and resentment that you had built up. (The liver is the place where the body primarily holds feelings of anger.) As you continue to twist your torso and breathe, first to one side and then to the other, you will notice how the pain in your stomach subsides and your feelings of resentment and anger become lighter as well.

Once you get your body back under control, then you will make better choices regarding your commitments to others as well as yourself.

35

Yoga Mudra

Yoga mudra is a sacred gesture that communicates the primal truth that all is *One*. The word mudra comes from the Sanskrit root "mud," which means to delight in. Mudra also means "seal" and generally relates to the hand gestures; however, in Hatha Yoga, mudra also relates to the physical body postures. These hand positions, and in particular this posture, controls the energy in the body. By folding our hands in the prayer position either at our heart or behind our back, we begin to feel more mentally focused. As we connect our hearts to our minds and then offer ourselves to our Divine Source in this posture, we begin to release ego and feel a more connected, unconditional sense of oneness with all that is.

> Behold, how good and how pleasant it is for brethren to dwell together in unity!
> —The Holy Bible, Psalms 133:1

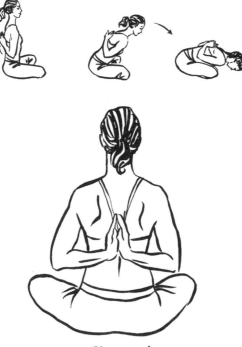

Yoga mudra.

It is through this feeling of "oneness" that we connect with our family and friends and to some extent, with co-workers and acquaintances. As we ask the question "How may I serve?" we lose the sense of separateness that our ego can develop which in turn provides for more loving and empowered relationships throughout our lives. Yoga mudra done in a yoga practice has far-reaching effects in our daily lives.

Empowerment Exercise: Yoga Mudra

Yoga Mudra Affirmation: *Humbly I bow to the Divine inside and outside of me. I seek only the TRUTH.*

This is one of those postures that many people may refer to as "being a pretzel." If you're not as flexible as you would like to be, don't let this asana deter you from trying it and feeling the transcendent benefits it offers. There are variations to this pose that will support different body types. I have listed the variations for this pose in the section on Cautions.

1. To practice this asana, sit on the floor (or your mat) with your legs crossed in lotus position. (Depending on your flexibility, a simple crossed leg position may be used instead of full lotus.)

2. Roll your shoulders back and downward as if you are pulling the bottom tips of your shoulder blades together.

3. Bring your hands together in the prayer position (anjali mudra) behind your back. Tuck in your stomach to help support the back. Be careful not to arch your lower back.

4. Inhale deeply, and as you exhale, fold forward bringing your forehead to rest on the floor. Continue breathing in a deep and regular inhalation/exhalation.

5. Your eyes can remain open or closed, but keep your mental gaze at the point between your eyes. Relax into this posture for about 4–8 breaths or as long as you feel comfortable and supported.

6. To release from the postures, bring your awareness to your stomach and strengthen it, supporting your lower back. Pull your shoulders down your back as you lift your torso upward and back to your seated position.

7. Gently release your hands from behind your back and place your prayer hands at your forehead for at least one full breath, then rest your hands either in your lap or on your knees, palms facing upward.

Benefits

Because yoga mudra is a forward bend, it is a calming and centering posture. It soothes the nervous system and induces a feeling of deep peace and tranquility. It also is a powerful way to internalize awareness and enhance the ability to surrender.

This posture cultivates contentment and inner peace while helping to release feelings of insecurity and fear. Because the shoulders and chest are open, this also stimulates the heart center, which releases feelings of love, compassion, and kindness.

On a physical level, yoga mudra massages the abdominal and pelvic organs as you breathe. It can also tone a sluggish liver and increase circulation. It is good for improving peristalsis and to relieve constipation.

Cautions

If you are unable to keep the palms of the hands together in prayer position behind your back without discomfort in your wrists or shoulders, bring your hands to your heart instead. The lotus leg position is the full extent of this pose; however, lotus can be difficult for many of us. You may sit in a simple crossed-leg position to practice this asana.

There are no major contraindications to this posture if you move into it with your own body's capabilities in mind. However, if you have shoulder or wrist problems and/or have had surgery on these areas, it is advisable that you do not place your hands behind your back, but do the variation with hands to heart.

Peace is a daily, a weekly, a monthly process, gradually changing opinions, slowly eroding old barriers, quietly building new structures.
—John F. Kennedy, former president of the United States

Real Life

The person who shared this story has honored me by allowing her experiences to be presented in this book. She asked to remain anonymous, however, so I respect her wishes.

"I went through a terrible breakup with a man whom I thought was my soul mate. We had been close friends for many years before our romance and I had felt such a kindred spirit with him throughout our relationship. Our spiritual paths were very similar, as were our hobbies and careers. To make a long story short, in my mind, we fit together so well that I believed we were meant to be together for the rest of our lives.

Very unexpectedly, he approached me one day and said he wanted to break up and told me he loved me but didn't feel he could be what I needed. No amount of my begging, rationalizing, nor sobbing could convince him otherwise and we parted ways because of his choice.

In the months that followed I struggled with depression over the loss I felt and feared that I would never find love like I had known with him. Also during that time I continued my yoga practice, as it was the only solid thing I felt I could hold on to.

At first I would practice yoga mudra as if pleading with God to bring him back to me. At times I would just fall into a heap and cry like a lost child. I continued to do yoga every day, even if I only managed to do one or two postures. However, I always did yoga mudra.

One morning, as I was folding into yoga mudra (the tears were gone but were replaced with a deep emptiness) I felt something flutter in my chest. It made me catch my breath and then my whole body relaxed. A feeling of release and complete unconditional love came over me so powerfully that I began to cry, but this time it wasn't from desperation but from feeling true love. It was bigger than I have ever felt before and I didn't even have a person to direct it to. That emotion was so powerful that I immediately came out of the pose and sat there trying to understand what had just happened to me.

In the days following, and as I continued to practice yoga mudra, I realized that my heart felt lighter and my thoughts were centered more around contentment and understanding rather than sorrow. I was beginning to let go of my feelings of loss and replace them with compassion for myself and an understanding and kindness toward my lost soul mate. Anger and fear were releasing from my body and emotions and my life was filling with more love and I began to have a brighter outlook on my future.

I truly believe it was yoga mudra that pierced through the grief and sadness in my heart and showed me how connected I am to all that is."

Empowerment Journal

Take a few moments now to write in your journal of the feelings you felt as you practiced yoga mudra. List everything you can think of from the physical aspects of the pose to the emotions it brought up and the mental thoughts.

Was it easy for you to fold into the pose or did you find tightness in your shoulders and wrists? Did your hips support you as you folded forward? If you chose to use the variations of the pose, how did that feel?

Did you notice your thoughts calming down or did you feel a flood of emotions? Perhaps you surrendered easily into that centered, calm place. In any event, write it all down and refer to your journal periodically to recount your practice of this pose and to notice your progress.

The following empowerment journal excerpt is from one of my students. This was his first class with me at a time in his life when he wanted to get healthy and find a more peaceful way of living. Reggie, I honor you!

I learned a lot in class today. Mainly I learned that I have never taken a real yoga class before. I have just been in exercise sessions that did not open up any areas and did not concentrate on holding a position and breathing like we did tonight. We held and stretched one area at a time and then would relax everything else ... very unusual feeling. We concentrated on breathing through the whole posture, releasing more as we exhaled. As we relaxed one side, I could actually feel it was open and the other side was not. To make a long story short, I loved the session and will continue to go back to class.

Mantras for Daily Living

If you need to slow down a bit, relax, and bring more focus, choose a slower mantra, one that you can recite at a slower pace and that does not have a rushed feel to it. I find that repeating the sound "OM" in a steady, rhythmic voice has one of the most profound and centering effects I have ever felt. When I am chanting "OM," there is no conflict within my heart nor am I concerned about any future events. "OM" keeps me grounded fully in the present moment. It is also good to chant "OM" while sitting in yoga mudra, as it reinforces the reverence of the posture and connects you with the universal pulse of the Cosmos.

The great and glorious masterpiece of man is to know how to live to purpose.
—Montaigne, translated by W.C. Hazlett (English essayist)

Here are a few sample mantras that you can choose from that relate to discipline and the empowerment of your dharma. Sample these and try your own, too. It is important to resonate with your mantra even if you do not concentrate on the words as you chant them.

- "SAT" ("I Am").
- "I express my discipline with my intention to stay present in each moment."
- "Intention plus right action equals discipline."
- "I trust that my dharma is revealed to me daily."
- "My yoga practice leads me to my dharma."

Dharma Discovery: Defining Your Life Purpose

Write down these two questions in your journal:

1. If I already had everything that I needed and desired, what would I do?
2. How am I best suited to serve the world?

In the highest sense, work is meant to be the servant of man, not the master ... what is vitally important is our attitude toward that work.
—Edmund Bordeaux Szekely, philosopher

After you've jotted down these questions, begin to answer them as thoughts come to you. You may write down ideas that come to you off the top of your head, but take your time to really consider your answers because some of them may be hidden behind your "have to's."

Try doing some of your favorite yoga poses with the intention of them revealing the answers to your questions about dharma. As you practice, ask yourself what activities give you joy and empowerment. Which ones open your heart? When do you feel truly alive? Is your practice, right now, helping to answer your questions for you? If you would still do what you are currently doing, then you are in your dharma because you have passion for what you do and you are expressing your talents.

For example, as I do my morning yoga and meditation routine, I can feel my body and mind wake up from my night of sleep and come alive to the new day. My thoughts do not rush ahead of me to all the things I have to do, but they rest in the pleasure of waking up and "being" in my body. I realize a deep contentment within myself without having to prove my actions to anyone, especially to myself. In that simple, peaceful place of breath where I am alone with my Self, I know that my life is on track and I am following my dharma. There is no resistance in my mind nor in my emotional body. I trust my intuition. It is in that serenity that I have realized my dharma for the day and for my life.

Maybe you've tried every kind of job there is from retail sales to food service to computer repair and you still feel unfulfilled in your life. How do you know what you're best suited for? The answers are simple and straightforward if you listen to your heart and your intuition. Do what brings you joy, whether it's babysitting for your grandkids, taking that job at the homeless shelter so you can help folks who are down on their luck, or managing a large corporation that specializes in environmental health. The point is, do what you love and the dharma will follow. You *will* be of service to others.

You get the idea, so get going. Make your list, practice your favorite yoga postures and discover what your true Self is trying to show you. Your dharma is waiting to be realized!

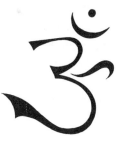

Chapter Three

Navigating the Twists and Turns of Life

As I sat down to write this chapter, I contemplated what it really means to navigate the twists and turns of life. Are we really caught in a raging river of experiences over which we have no control? Or do all of our experiences come to us from choices we have made before now? I think, perhaps, it is a little of both. We do create our own reality with the choices we make and thoughts we think; however, since we in human consciousness cannot know the motivations of all action, we seem to be caught off guard, so to speak, with much of what life has to offer. We live our lives through our own realities and perceptions, which sometimes can be misleading. It is with these thoughts that I contemplate the twists and turns of living.

we live life in our own reality –) can be misleading

Let your heart's light guide you to my house.
Let your heart's light show you that we are one.
—Rumi, poet

To navigate means to walk, or find one's way. We are finding our way through the challenges and accomplishments of our lives, but how? What best serves us as we maneuver our bodies, minds, and emotions through our daily existence? There is no exact way for us to follow; however, there are universal practices that have been handed down through the ages that each of us develops and incorporates into our lives as we see fit.

There are many things that we use as guides to support our emotional and mental bodies, such as contemplation, study and research, spiritual reading, participating in psychotherapy or self-help groups, or even biofeedback and meditation. Physically, we jog and lift weights, we swim, hike, and play various sports, and we even occasionally allow ourselves massage and physical therapy when we've overdone our training. But there is one cohesive, all-encompassing activity we do that integrates all of our self-help activities and unites us with our soul, our true Self. For many of us yoga is the compass with which we use to guide us through our lives.

Each of us finds a unique and varied approach to our own life. This approach in the yogic tradition is called *sadhana*. The disciplines of yoga, meditation, service, self-study, and devotion are a few of the spiritual practices that help us to reach toward enlightenment and a clearer understanding of our existence on earth. For most of us, a combination of practices is how we best approach our spiritual discipline of sadhana.

For some people, emphasis on a vigorous physical training is the most important aspect of their sadhana, while others prefer a more mental approach with study and contemplation on subjects relating to their dharma (see Chapter 2). Still others prefer a more devotional and service-oriented way of living life. All of these approaches are embodied in the many different paths of yoga and can be "mixed and matched" to shape our life practice, but ultimately we find there is one major form we follow and we intersperse aspects of the other approaches.

As I have studied and lived yoga throughout the years, I have come to realize that my main approach is through physical practice and devotion, yet I do incorporate service to others and deeper study. For example, my daily routine consists of morning meditation and contemplation followed with physical yoga postures. Sometimes I will do the postures first if my body and heart advise in that direction. As I move through my daily activities, I find great joy in teaching yoga classes and even assisting people in other areas of life. Part of my evenings are spent again with meditation and a few restorative yoga poses to bring me back to my center. For me, this is my sadhana, the practice I use to help me navigate the twists and turns of my life. Sadhana requires dedication and devotion to yourself and to your higher Self. When you can devote focused time to your personal practice, you will become empowered in every aspect of your life. If you allow sadhana to be the foundation of the way you approach your life, you will see its positive, empowering results on your mat as well.

Ask yourself what feels most comfortable in your life. What type of yoga do you gravitate toward the most: physical, devotional, study, service? What style do you prefer? Do you find that you gravitate toward a slower, gentler routine or do you prefer vinyasa, constantly flowing from one posture to the next? Once you can determine how you best approach your practice on the mat, you will then begin to deepen it. In turn, your yoga practice will filter into your reality showing you healthier, more enlightened ways of approaching your life.

Sadhana

*discipline
*self-study
*surrender

Sadhana is the Sanskrit term for "realizing." In yoga, it refers to the path one takes in their life to achieve awareness. Disciplined action, self-study, and surrender to God constitute the practice of yoga. Your sadhana is a personal collection of disciplines, making up your spiritual practice that leads you to Self-realization.

> Yoga is a potent antidote to suffering (duhkha) and, if consistently practiced, can fulfill our deep-seated impulse toward inner freedom, peace of mind and lasting happiness.
>
> —Georg Feuerstein, founder-director of Yoga Research and Education Center

Sadhana is different for each individual who dedicates his or her life to spiritual awareness; however, it is useless if not practiced with sincerity. It is not enough to merely give lip service to what you hope to accomplish with your practice, but you have to make effort in the right direction. As Patanjali has stated in his timeless writings of the Yoga Sutras, discipline provides the energy; self-study serves as the road map; and pure awareness is the destination.

What form of discipline are you using to navigate the road map of your life? It is important to have a guideline, whether it is a formally written list, or an embodied sense of who you are and how you live. This guideline allows you to evaluate your experiences in life so that you can build on their teachings and plot your course toward greater awareness and enlightenment. Keep in mind, however, that your guidelines should not be rigid and unchangeable, but they should be fluid and have the ability to change as you do.

 guideline should be flexible

Daily Spiritual Practice

When we think of a spiritual practice, we may consider going to a church or synagogue, saying prayers, and following the traditions of a particular faith that we subscribe to. Yes, this is a spiritual practice if done with intention and devotion. But your whole life can be a spiritual practice as well.

> Let us try to recognize the precious nature of each day.
> —His Holiness the 14th Dalai Lama, Tenzin Gyatso

Taking a closer look at your daily life, you will see that each breath you take and action you take can become part of what brings awareness and a sense of "holy" to your life.

Last winter I saw a couple of doves perched on my back stoop. As I silently watched the pair, I wondered how they felt about commitment, knowing that doves mate for life. As I related their simple, yet profound connection to my own relationship to life, my friends, and my work, I was able to see the spiritual teaching they offered me in their own connection to being. Birds (and animals) don't seek, nor research, nor practice ... they just "live" in a state of "being." Ah, my spiritual lesson for the day was given! Just "be" and all that is shall be revealed to me in the perfect time. Sometimes our spiritual practice can be as simple and profound as that.

Think of an example in your own life when a small, almost insignificant event made a profound impact on the way you view your own spirituality. Did you feel as if a light bulb went on inside your head, or did you feel it more as a knowing deep inside your heart? Either way, it's often the small things that make a big impact in our lives and to our spiritual practice. This is not to say that epoch events cannot change us and deepen our spiritual awareness, but to remember that you have opportunities every day to achieve enlightenment through your spiritual search.

Right now, at this moment, take a break from whatever it is you are doing and either sit up or stand up straight, feeling strong in your bones yet relaxed in your muscles. Inhale deeply and just when you think you can't fill your lungs any further, breathe in a little more. Hold your breath for one count and then exhale. As you reach the end of your exhale, breathe out even more, push it out, and then feel the pause in between breaths before you continue with another inhale.

Practice this expanded breathing technique for as long as you feel comfortable and notice what happens to you physically, emotionally, and mentally. Does your chest feel expanded and fuller? Do you feel light-headed and/or feel any emotions coming to the surface of your consciousness?

As you bring your breath back to normal inhalations and exhalations, place your awareness on the most prominent feeling that you are experiencing, whether it is physical, emotional, or mental, and notice the new understandings you are coming to.

Acts of Accomplishment

Our society is seemingly obsessed with success. We usually measure our levels of success by achievements, such as powerful positions in business, gaining large sums of money, and enjoying a degree of fame. It seems, though, that these accomplishments don't have all we need to make us truly fulfilled and happy human beings.

obsession w. success + money

What, then, is the true definition of "accomplishment"? *Webster's* dictionary gives a beautiful definition of what it truly is. Accomplishment is an act or instance of carrying into effect, fulfillment. It is something that is done admirably and credibly. What does that mean in the spiritual sense? The term "right action" comes to mind as I contemplate the true meaning of accomplishment. A job well done, no matter how insignificant to the world it may seem, is an accomplishment. And when that job is done with reverence and intention, it becomes part of our spiritual practice. The fact that we actually "show up" to our lives, whether we are noticed for good deeds or not, is important; however, we may feel that we have failed when we do not achieve what our peers define as success.

Do you have a friend who is financially well off and is constantly traveling and buying new things while you work long hours every day just to make ends meet? Do you compare your life to hers? How does it make you feel? If you are judging your life by the things she does have and the things you don't have, I would bet that you are feeling like you haven't accomplished much in your life.

How can we enjoy our worldly successes and not identify ourselves with them? Learning to have perspective about others' successes and our successes and failures is important. The only real success in life is living with an open and loving heart in our truth.

This can be applied to yoga. Think of when you started to practice yoga for the first time. Perhaps you are at that point now. What is your self-talk saying to you? Does it admonish you for even trying something new, or worse yet, "strange"? Do you entertain thoughts of "it's too hard" or "I could never do that"? Maybe you judge yourself for not knowing how to practice yoga before you've even had your first lesson.

It is important to realize that you are not your inabilities nor failures. You are not even your successes. You are a spiritual being who uses the experiences of your accomplishments and failures to know yourself more deeply.

Think of a yoga pose that you have been having difficulty with. What are your challenges with this pose? Is your balance shaky, are your muscles too tight, or do you need more strength before you can support a certain pose? Whatever your challenge, come to this asana with a sense of acceptance and be open to learn what this pose has to teach you. Continue to practice even though you may lose your balance or not have enough strength to hold the posture for more than a second or two. Release yourself from the act of accomplishment and surrender into "being" the pose. It is in the letting go of the achievement that we accomplish true success. Likewise, this is true for our life.

Your yoga practice and your daily life are intertwined, in that one will always show you examples of how it can affect the other. An accomplishment on the mat transfers to your accomplishments in real life. For example, if you have been working on balancing postures and you find that you are able to stand in Vrkasana (Tree Pose) without wobbling for longer than a minute, you may start to notice that your life reflects more balance. You may see it in the way you manage your time, in the amount of money you are able to save, and even in the quality of relationships that you choose to be a part of.

You can clearly see how your beliefs and perspectives of achievement affect your yoga practice as well. If you come to your mat with an open heart and a willingness to surrender to what is, you will find that your postures are more solid and your body is more fluid. If you honestly examine your life and your yoga practice, you can find many examples of accomplishment.

Living with Impermanence

Why is impermanence so difficult for us to accept? Perhaps it is because we have a fear of the unknown or of losing out. This comes back to the realization that nothing can be relied on to stay the same. Impermanence is the very essence of reality. That being said, it is futile to hold on to attachments, either of the mind or of the body.

> Impermanence is a principle of harmony. When we don't struggle against it, we are in harmony with reality.
>
> —Pema Chodron, Buddhist nun and teacher

Think of a moment when you felt exquisitely alive; the kind of moment you wished would last forever. Standing by a magnificent waterfall, trembling on the edge of a first kiss, sleeping under the stars, immersing yourself in a project or sport, the high of standing on a mountaintop and gazing out on an expansive horizon, the glory of a red and purple and gold sunset. As you recall those times, or others that seem more vivid to you, remember how present you were in the moment. You let go of the concepts you had of past and future, even if it was for a few minutes, and you surrendered to and accepted the "now." Do you remember how free and alive you felt during those times? Inevitably, though, the desire to hold on to those moments turned them into attachments and wants. You no longer felt the freedom of just being in the moment.

Contrast that to moments when you were caught in the insanity of rush-hour traffic, a workday morning when you were running late, a hurried lunch so you could get a dozen papers off your desk, and a frazzled evening doing laundry and paying bills. Did you feel pressured and stifled? Were you holding on to fear and frustration from the situations you felt stuck in? Was a sense of impending doom looming over you in those moments of chaos, and did you wish life was all over?

These are examples of the inability to accept impermanence in your life. When we can understand and accept that neither we nor the people, places, and events in our lives stay the same, then we come to accept impermanence.

Acknowledge impermanence when your life feels difficult so you won't be overburdened with your challenges, but remember it too when things are going well, so that you will stay present enough to relish the sweet moments of "now" in your life. Know that nothing is permanent but change.

A friend of mine in Denver, Colorado, used to comment on the constantly changing weather. On a day in the middle of January we would be enjoying a balmy 70 degrees and then turn around the very next afternoon and have to shovel six inches of snow off the sidewalk! He would say, "Don't like the weather? Stick around for an hour, it's bound to change!" Ah, the beautiful lesson of impermanence is so eloquently expressed in that statement! If we can surrender to change, we can unlock the feelings of fear and loss that create suffering, and transform them to a deeper understanding of Self in the present moment. When we can accept the impermanence of life and release fear of the unknown, we empower ourselves with surrender. I don't mean that we "give up" through surrender; rather, we open ourselves to all possibilities and we are empowered to achieve all of our dreams and desires.

For the next week, make a commitment to yourself to practice a yoga pose that you particularly don't like or find hard to do. Perhaps your hamstrings are tight and you really don't like Paschimotanasana (Seated Forward Bend). Every day for the next week, give yourself over to this asana rather than force yourself to do it. Surrender your preconceived thoughts about your body and open yourself to the possibility of change. Start where you are with your body and spend time here, concentrating on the fullness of your breath and its ability to move you deeper into the pose. When you feel you have had enough, release from the posture and continue with your day.

Each time you come back to this pose, notice if there are any differences. Can you bend farther forward without discomfort? Do your legs stay flat on the floor? Have you been able to release any feelings, insecurity, and resistance? Perhaps your thoughts are turning from "I can't" to "I am."

This weeklong journey is revealing how change occurs and also how important impermanence is to our spiritual growth and higher awareness.

Practice: "Letting Go"

Lie on your back with your knees bent and bring the soles of your feet together, heels and toes touching. Allow your knees to drop out like a butterfly. Let your arms rest at your sides, palms facing upward to help open the shoulders. Breathe into this open posture for about five minutes and notice what sensations come up for you.

All is change. All yields its place and goes.
—Euripides, Greek playwright

This yoga posture is called Supta Baddha Konasana, which I frequently use in my classes to instill the feelings of surrender and letting go in my students.

As you recline in this pose, you may feel as if you want to put your hands on your abdomen or bring your knees together. It may be difficult for you to surrender your knees to gravity and let them relax out to your sides. As you try to force surrender or push those feelings of discomfort away, you may find that you become more agitated. Breathe into those feelings; stay with them.

Keep your mind engaged with the agitation until you gain the perspective that through your holding on, you are having unpleasant experiences. What would happen if you let go, and surrendered into the openness of this pose? This is how you engage in life, by accepting the sensations and situations as they are and letting go.

Letting go is one of the most frequently studied practices of yoga, yet it is one of the most difficult to understand. Also referred to as detachment or surrender, it tends to make us feel uncomfortable at the thought of "losing control" or being vulnerable. This is a misunderstanding of the concept of letting go. What are we really losing, anyway? In surrendering to the present moment, the only thing you may lose would be the fear of the future and the regrets of the past.

When you allow yourself to be in the moment and see things as they truly are, then you can love yourself and others without hidden attachments. Detachment is the greatest act of love. When you let go, you are able to see the truth that has been with you the whole time.

Ardha Matsyendrasana (Half Spinal Twist)

As the name suggests, Ardha Matsyendrasana twists the spine to achieve deep physical, mental, and emotional benefits. Twisting poses are cooling and rejuvenating. When done properly, they loosen and stretch the full length of the spine, helping to release tension in all aspects of our awareness.

Watch me be a pretzel, Auntie!
—Payton Joyce Wood, yogini and my 9-year-old niece (*yogini* is the term for a female yoga practitioner)

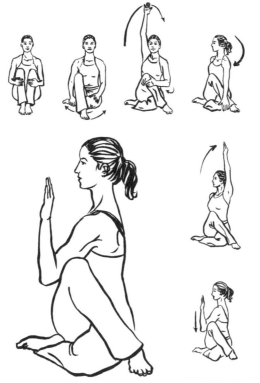

Ardha Matsyendrasana (Half Spinal Twist).

Along with the physiological benefits of Ardha Matsyendrasana comes the powerful stimulation of your power center. Remember the third chakra, your solar plexus and power center? As you move through the half spinal twist, not only are you lengthening and energizing your spine, but you are squeezing and flushing the organs of your belly which in turn, cleanses any "stuck" energy in that area. Upon finishing this pose you may feel more self-confident and powerful.

Empowerment Exercise: Ardha Matsyendrasana

Ardha Matsyendrasana Affirmation: *I am resilient to the changes in my life. I welcome the unknown.*

Twisting postures are essential for a complete yoga practice and must always be included in any balanced routine, but they can also be done alone as needed. Try this posture when you need that extra boost of personal power and self-confidence.

1. Begin with knees bent close to the body and slide your left foot under your right knee, placing it on the floor to the outside of your right hip. Make sure your left knee is directly in front of your navel.

2. Place your right foot on the outside of your left knee on the floor. Sit evenly on both sitbones.

3. Reach your right arm forward and make a circle, rotating the shoulder to the right as you place your right hand on the floor directly behind your right hip.

4. Raise the left arm up and then bend the elbow and place it on the outside of the right thigh. (If you are unable to place the left elbow to the outside of the right thigh, you can wrap the left arm around the right knee.)

5. Inhale and lengthen your spine as you press down through your right arm to support the twist.

6. On the exhalation, pull your belly in and gently rotate from the lower back. Make sure that your neck and shoulders do not lead the twist, but you are fully mobile and supported from your lumbar spine (the lower back).

7. To exit the pose, inhale and lengthen your spine. Then, begin to rotate back toward your center as you exhale. Continue to support your lower back with your stomach muscles.

8. Repeat to other side.

Benefits

The benefits of twisting are numerous, with varied effects throughout the body, but the asanas must be performed with correct posture so as not to compress and injure the spine.

Ardha Matsyendrasana, and spinal twists in general, are beneficial for people who sit or stand for long periods of time. The "squeeze and soak" effect of the twist helps to move the fluids of the body (such as blood, spinal fluid, and lymph) through their proper pathways to enrich you with fresh oxygen and prana (life force). It also encourages the discs of the spine to absorb fluid, which enables them to maintain a full and plump shape in order to support the spinal column.

Through this physiological process, Ardha Matsyendrasana increases elasticity of the spine, shoulders, and neck while strengthening the internal and external oblique muscles. It also helps to relax emotional tension in the chest and helps to release rigidity throughout the body and mind.

This pose is not only good for the muscular and structural systems of the body, but positively affects the internal organs and systems as well. Spinal twisting improves digestion and peristalsis. Through the "squeeze/soak" effect, the kidneys, liver, gall bladder, spleen, and pancreas are all oxygenated and massaged.

On an emotional level, Ardha Matsyendrasana helps to cultivate the heart qualities such as compassion, kindness, generosity, and unconditional love by opening the shoulders and stretching across the chest. For instance, if you have been sad or depressed, practice this pose and notice how you feel immediately afterwards. Most likely your emotions will have stabilized and you will be less reactive.

Cautions

Even considering how wonderful spinal twists are for your total well-being, there are still some things to be cautious about. Always remember that every body is unique, which makes it very important that you listen to your body and practice this asana according to how you feel.

Never apply too much leverage to your twisting motions and make sure you are not swaying your lower back. It is important to remember to pull the navel toward the spine to help strengthen the lower back during the twist.

A final word of caution to those who have had spinal and rib injuries and/or hip replacements/dislocations: Check with your doctor for advice before doing this pose. There are variations that you can do if this particular asana creates too much stress on your body.

Laughter is not at all a bad beginning for a friendship, and it is far the best ending for one.

—Oscar Wilde, English poet, playwright, and novelist

Real Life

While interviewing friends and students for their real-life yoga stories, my friend Mickey shared his experience of spontaneous yoga.

"This was during a time in my life when I was doing a lot of yoga and was in great physical shape. I was doing stuff like Scorpion and Handstand ... all kinds of poses.

I was with a bunch of my friends one evening and we were sitting around just goofing off and laughing and acting strange as we could do so well when we got on the subject of yoga. Most of my friends didn't do yoga and certainly didn't know how good it could make you feel, so I jumped off the couch and sat down on the floor and started doing a Half Spinal Twist to give them an idea of what yoga looked like.

They all started laughing at me and then all of a sudden I could feel a total energy release in myself and in the room! It made me feel so happy. It was as if this amazing shivering light was shooting up my spine. I would twist and all of a sudden my body felt ... ah, so good. There was an incredible release of tension throughout my spine and the muscles just relaxed.

I felt a release in my nervous system, too, and I couldn't help laughing with all my friends. It's like it made them all giddy and then I couldn't tell if they were laughing at me or with me. Whatever was happening, it sure felt good to me, and everyone in the room seemed to really be having a good time.

I guess the best way I could describe the feeling for myself is a physical utopia. The muscles twisting like that on both sides increased the blood so much … it was a great feeling. It took me out of my body and into the feeling. It didn't feel like I was in my body, but felt more like my body became the feeling. Light, joy, feelings of well-being … all that describes my experience in Half Spinal Twist (Ardha Matsyendrasana).

Even though I haven't been doing as much yoga as back then, I can still vividly remember how it energized me and filled me with such a great feeling.

Hmmm, come to think of it, maybe I do need to do more yoga now!"

Empowerment Journal

Take some time now to write in your journal of how you felt as you practiced Ardha Matsyendrasana. What were your thoughts, if any were moving through your mind? List all the physical sensations that you felt as well as the emotions it brought up for you. Did you notice any such feelings as joy, freedom, or happiness or did you feel any fear, or perhaps anger? List your thoughts, emotions, and physical abilities and/or challenges now.

Was this pose particularly easy for you or did you find it to be a challenge? In what way was it easy? In what way was it difficult? Sometimes a posture can be easy to do physically but our emotions or thoughts may want to rebel against how we "feel" in the pose. Other times an asana may be difficult to execute; however, we are so emotionally empowered to practice that the pose itself becomes stronger through our mental and emotional support.

Remember you don't have to spend hours writing in your journal. Sometimes you may want to jot down a few notes and other times you may spend quite some time evaluating and processing. It all depends on how each posture affects you at any given time in your life. Things change, so keep in mind that what you are feeling today with Ardha Matsyendrasana may be a completely different experience from what you will feel while performing this asana later.

Here is an example journal entry from an anonymous student:

... in a hurry today but felt drawn to do some twisting. I sat down and did a simple twist and it didn't feel deep enough so I moved into the Half Spinal Twist. Oh boy, that did it! Even though my back started feeling better because I needed the stretch, I started to feel unsure of myself. Today's the day I'm supposed to find out if I get this new job ... and I really need it. I just kept breathing and backed out of it a little bit. I started to feel better.

Mantras for Daily Living

The following mantras are related to "letting go" and the art of accomplishing. They can be good tools to help keep you focused in your sadhana, or your spiritual practice; however, if these do not resonate with you, your own mantra may better serve you. Surrender your heart to what motivates your inner voice, choose your mantra and chant it, vibrating it throughout your entire being.

- "This too shall pass."
- "I embrace change and let go of fear."
- "Letting go of the past releases me to new possibilities."
- "Because I live in the 'now' I can accomplish great things."
- "I am perfect just the way I am."

Sometimes it's all I can do to just keep saying "help me God!"
—Helen Wood, my mother and teacher

Try using a faster mantra to generate energy and overcome dullness in your life. You may even choose to recite a fast mantra while doing a morning yoga practice to jump-start your day so that you have a greater supply of focus and energy to support all that you have to accomplish.

For example, you might choose one word or phrase like "energy" or "life is good" and repeat it quickly during your morning yoga practice. If you find yourself in a rush in the mornings and can't find the time for a full yoga practice, try standing in Tadasana (Mountain Pose, see Chapter 1) and chant "life is good" as you breathe in and raise your arms over your head. As you exhale, lower your arms and repeat "life is good." Repeat this mantra and the action of Tadasana for as long as you are comfortable. Once you complete it, notice the focus, energy, and positive thoughts you have just instilled in yourself.

Putting Your Spiritual Practice Together

One of our human goals is to increase happiness and reduce pain and suffering in our lives. Underlying this fundamental reality is the desire to find our true identity, our true Self.

The quest for certainty blocks the search for meaning. Uncertainty is the very condition to impel man to unfold his powers.
—Erich Fromm, American psychoanalyst and philosopher

Yoga is one of the many forms of enlightenment that wakes us up to this ongoing quest so that we become aware of the reasons why we are here on this earth. Through physical, emotional, and mental practices, we seek to achieve an understanding of who we are and how we accomplish our purpose in this life. Sadhana is a form of spiritual discipline, referred to as the path to Realization. It encompasses all forms of yoga and meditation as well as self-study and surrender to reach Self-realization.

Self-realization, then, is the recovery of our true identity through applying discernment to everything that comes into our lives. The Self does not necessarily equal the actions and events of our lives, but transcends them. In other words, our spiritual practice is not who we are, but is the tool we use to realize who we are. Through self-inspection with the physical practice of yoga, we can accomplish transcendence through the realization of impermanence.

It is the realization of impermanence, the understanding that everything changes, that allows us to let go of our attachments to the past and release our fears of an unknown future, and live more fully in the present moment.

We have so many ways in which to reach our spiritual potential, but how do we decide which techniques and philosophies are the ones that best suit us? Let us, in this timeless moment of the now, choose how we approach our spiritual discipline. Discover what resonates with you, whether it is a physical workout, meditation practices, or a combination of the many different approaches to yoga. Let your sadhana bring you closer to the realization of who you really are.

Part Two

Finding Your Path to Empowerment: Patanjali's Eight-Limbed Path

In this part we will discuss Patanjali's Eight-Limbed Path, which yogis follow to reach enlightenment. In the scriptures of the Yoga Sutras, the eight steps to enlightenment build on each other to help the yoga practitioner achieve liberation from the senses and thus reach samadhi, or spiritual enlightenment.

Chapter 4 focuses on the power of love and encompasses the first step of moral restraint along our eight-fold path. Chapter 5 takes us to the second step and discusses the observances a yogi must take to heart along his or her path to enlightenment. Chapter 6 moves up the path to our third step, which is probably the most understood by many yoga practitioners. We will discuss the practice of Hatha Yoga and how it affects our mind/body/spirit connection.

Chapter 7 encompasses the fourth step to enlightenment by expanding awareness to our breath. Pranayama is the breathing aspect of Hatha Yoga, which leads us further toward liberation. Chapter 8 celebrates our journey on this path, stepping us to the fifth limb of turning inward, pratyahara. In this chapter we begin to trust our intuition. Chapters 9 through 11 coincide with each other in that the last three steps on our path to enlightenment are inner-connected. Concentration, meditation, and integration all work to create the ultimate of transformations, liberation. Finally, Chapter 12 shows us how, by following the Eight-Limbed Path, we experience an empowered life full of joy, discovery, and possibilities.

Let us take this journey, step by step, and uncover our own unlimited potential to create and live an empowered life through the practice of yoga on and off our mat.

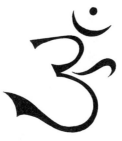

Chapter Four

Compassion: The Essence of Real Love

Love is a many splendored thing. We have all experienced it throughout our lives. It comes in many forms and faces—from the nurturing support of our parents, to the kindred connection of a best friend, to the unconditional devotion of our life partner. Especially, we come to know love through the acceptance and inner awareness of our self.

Many texts and philosophies have stated that we cannot accept nor understand real love of another person until we find that love within ourselves. How, then, do we know what real love is? Through the practice of yoga and especially the ten moral principles explained in Patanjali's Yoga Sutras, we come to know that our true nature is love. By following the guidelines of the yamas, which I'll discuss in this chapter, and niyamas, which I'll explain in Chapter 5, we gain a better understanding of the essence of real love and how it applies to our internal self as well as our external interactions.

[handwritten margin notes] essence of love →internal self →others

The Five Moral Restraints (Yamas)

Little is known about the life of Patanjali, one of India's most famed sages, but his body of work, the Yoga Sutras, has become a foundational practice for which much of yoga is based. There are eight aspects, known as "limbs," of Patanjali's practical spirituality. One limb builds upon the other. The eight-fold path has been referred to as a ladder leading from common existence and self-absorption to Self-realization beyond the ego. The practices of the yamas (and niyamas) have been referred to as "eternal religion" because they represent the core teachings of all major religions. These eight limbs will be discussed further in the following pages of this book.

Yoga is based on a foundation of universal ethics, and the first limb therefore is not of postures or meditation, but of moral discipline, the yamas. The yamas should not be thought of as rigid commandments, but as skillful ways of realizing true love and living in the world without increasing its suffering or our own. The yamas include five important moral obligations:

- Non-harming (ahimsa)
- Non-stealing (asteya)
- Chastity (brahmacharya)
- Non-attachment (aparigraha)
- Truthfulness (satya)

The yamas are referred to as the external disciplines because they are the ways we aspire to live in this world. Through the yamas our actions are guided toward the benefit for all life. Practically speaking, the yamas benefit us as individuals, too. Each of these disciplines increases our insight and brings us to equanimity by eliminating the distractions of the outside world. We make a vow to live our lives to a higher standard, seeking enlightenment.

Non-Harming

Ahimsa (non-harming) is the most fundamental of these moral codes and is translated to mean nonviolence in thought and deed. So what does this mean in regular words? In short, non-harming relates to everything in our lives, from the type of food we put into our bodies, to the way we talk to the grocery store clerk or our children or friends, to the way we treat the earth. Non-harming even refers to the way we talk to and treat ourselves. We do harm every time we attempt to sway someone to our point of view or even impress our will or beliefs onto others.

For example, you have a few errands to run while on your lunch break and you forgot to bring your lunch with you. You're starving but you have to get to the bank and the cleaners because you know there won't be any time after work. Already your stomach is growling as you rush through traffic at breakneck speed in order to accomplish everything in 60 minutes. You see a McDonald's and swing into the drive-thru to grab a soda, french fries, and a burger with the works and promptly tear into it as you drive down the road.

By the time you get back to the office, you have finished your "lunch on the run" and you've managed to take care of your errands. But you were rude to the clerk at the bank because she was taking too long, and you didn't even have time to smile at the man at the cleaners because you were in such a rush to get back to work.

Well, you didn't run over anyone, so how could ahimsa (non-harming) apply to you? Let's back up a little bit to the time when you actually started your lunch hour.

As I stated earlier, non-harming applies to you as well as others. In starting off your adventure in a rush, you created stress for yourself and compounded it by not having lunch to relieve your hunger. To make matters worse, you ate something that was unhealthy for your body and called it "lunch." You weren't even able to be conscious of what you were eating. The first person you harmed, then, was yourself.

Next, let's take a look at all the travelers on the road with you. In not driving carefully—and eating lunch as you drove—you created potential harm for yourself (again) and others, not to mention the poor bank clerk and the guy at the cleaners. One simple act on your part that could change the whole scenario would have been to prioritize your time and honor yourself. Perhaps you could have gone only to the bank and then stopped at the local market to pick up a salad or healthy sandwich. Once back at work, with time to spare, you could have enjoyed your lunch and then called your spouse to ask him or her to pick up the dry cleaning. Voilà! No more stress, you've taken care of yourself, and you were present with the people you talked to. Ahimsa at its finest.

Keep in mind that you are living the non-harming path every time you say a kind word to a stranger, or pick up litter, or even refrain from gossiping. Ahimsa has to be practiced not only through action but also in word and thought. It is the unconditional intention of goodwill toward all beings at all times and in all situations.

Let's apply this to our yoga practice. When you are breathing into a pose, allowing your body to move with your breath, you are living ahimsa. But when you force yourself into a posture and you feel pushed and tense, you have forgotten the non-harming path.

Look around you now and see if you can find ways of living ahimsa. Opportunities surround you. All you have to do is become aware of them and then act.

Non-Stealing

The second moral code of the yamas is non-stealing (asteya). Although the word non-stealing is self-explanatory, it is meant to be understood in a more comprehensive sense. Notice how this virtue relates to "Thou Shalt Not Covet," as laid out in the Ten Commandments. It's true that we should avoid any thought or action of stealing, but what is the root for our intentions of theft? Wanting what someone else has, coveting, is a form of jealousy. But where does jealousy come from?

Our external grasping after and taking of things (including relationships) that don't belong to us is an expression of fear. It is the ego's attempt to overcome its basic feelings of isolation. The ego's basic nature is that of separateness; therefore, it feels threatened by lack and will do whatever it can to feel larger and more important. When it perceives another as having more than itself, jealousy arises. In doing so, the ego intrudes into the lives of others as it selfishly tries to accommodate its own feeling of lack.

Stealing doesn't only mean taking property or coveting another person's relationship. It also includes being egotistical in relationship, which causes the other person to feel inadequate or hurt in some way through your words or actions. In a sense, you are stealing another person's self-confidence and dignity.

When we apply the virtue of non-stealing, we surrender our ego to our higher Self and have faith that we are ultimately and divinely provided for. We believe there is enough (of whatever we need) for everyone and

64

neutralize selfish exp. of ego

all things come to us in the right moment. In practicing abstention from greed and jealousy, we begin to neutralize the selfish expressions of the ego.

You may wonder how this virtue of non-stealing can be applied to your yoga class. It's simple: When you are working with your postures and seek only to express the fullness of each pose within yourself, you are practicing asteya (non-stealing). You are not looking at someone else and wishing you looked like them, or had their balance, or owned their yoga blanket. To the true student of yoga, nothing else matters except for the experiencing of yoga itself. Your thoughts are drawn more to your internal awareness and less on the external "things" that you feel you might be lacking. When you release your sense of want and desire and you can be fulfilled with what you have in each moment, then you are following the path of non-stealing.

Chastity

The dictionary definition of chastity is moral purity. The Sanskrit term for chastity, brahmacharya, literally means "brahmic conduct" and refers to living a life in moderation and with self-control. It is the attempt to break away from duality, the relationship between two alternatives existing in opposition to each other. Examples of duality are light and dark, day and night, male and female, yin and yang.

moderation
self-control

Because of the duality between male and female, those that follow the path of chastity refer to it as the structured practice of celibacy. Celibacy acts to release the distinction between male and female and to regard all people as the same, to ultimately transcend the bodily needs to attain the eternal Self and promote a deeper intimacy with all beings.

On the physical level, chastity involves the abstinence from sexual activity; however, some schools of yoga qualify this by explaining the principle of moderation with respect to one's personal life. For example, married yogis, or those in a committed relationship, practice brahmacharya by abstaining from casual sexual contact and sexual conversations with others. They restrict their sexuality to times of intimacy with their partner. This not only is spoken of in yogic texts, but can be found in other major religions of the world such as Christianity and Judaism.

There are definite ideas about what is considered legitimate sex and what is thought of as a waste of vital energy. Sexual exploitation is considered a waste in that it creates a type of violence and deception (referring to ahimsa) that does not honor the individuals involved.

Think of the many commercials that you and your family watch between your favorite TV shows. There are beautiful women, half-dressed, throwing their lovely manes of hair around as they try to sell you everything from make-up and shampoo to clothing and even new trucks! Have you noticed how the media spotlights sex either through tabloids or TV? These are all examples of exploitation. The sacredness and the true meaning are lost from the natural and physical bodily expressions of sex.

You might be asking, what does abstaining from sex have to do with my yoga practice? The act of abstaining helps to bring a deep clarity regarding your own sexuality and feelings. It makes you accountable to yourself and to others for the choices you make. Likewise, when you become more focused on your mat—more accountable for your practice instead of half-heartedly going through the motions—you gain clarity and insight into the workings of your physical body as well as your mind and emotions. It is through this clarity that you approach your life with respect and honor for not only yourself, but for all who share in your life.

Non-Attachment

The Sanskrit word *aparigraha* is the term for non-attachment or greedlessness. Its strict definition is the non-acceptance of gifts because they tend to generate attachment and the fear of loss. A more palpable way of looking at non-attachment is in living a life of simplicity. What Patanjali was trying to convey through this moral code of the Sutras is that we, as the eternal Self, are all that we will ever need and possessions only distract us from our true nature.

> In detachment lies the wisdom of uncertainty ... in the wisdom of uncertainty lies the freedom from the known .... And in our willingness to step into the unknown, we surrender ourselves to the creative mind that orchestrates the dance of the universe.
> —Deepak Chopra, best-selling author and physician

In our fear we have forgotten that we are already all that we need. Greed is the longing for things, material or not, especially a desire for more than what we need. It is the fear of not having enough of whatever you want—whether it's money, better romantic relationships, bigger cars, more proficiency in your yoga postures, or more recognition. The list could go on indefinitely. When we can live unattached to the "things" of the outside world and trust that we already have what we need and all will be provided in the time needed, we then release greed and fear and can approach our lives with contentment and peace.

The lesson of non-attachment doesn't always come easily because of our human conditioning. Especially during times of war in our country's history, we were taught to stock up on food and water and never to throw anything away because we might need it "someday." Although the concept of frugality promotes less waste, it can be taken too far and be termed as hoarding and selfishness. Fear of loss is the underlying emotion to these actions. When we loosen the grip on our fear and begin to trust in our eternal Selves, we then can more easily approach non-attachment.

Try practicing non-attachment while in your yoga practice. Is there a posture that you are intensely practicing because it is difficult and will make you feel strong and proud once you accomplish it? Do you practice so hard that you become frustrated and angry at times when you can't seem to hold the pose? Does it seem like the harder you practice, the more elusive the pose becomes? This is because you have become attached to the outcome of how you will look and feel in regard to your ego. Try taking a few deep breaths and let go of your image of how you are "supposed" to feel and look in this particular asana. Take a break from practicing this pose, whether it's a few moments or a few days. When you come back to it, approach it with beginner's mind, as if you are seeing it for the first time. Tell yourself that you will achieve this posture when the time is right to do so and then begin without expectation.

Nature is such a beautiful example of living with non-attachment. Notice how the earth changes with the seasons, never holding on to one longer than the other. Trees bud in the spring and their leaves grow to fullness in the summer. They let go of their leaves in the fall to stand naked in the winter months only to repeat the cycle. There is an inherent wisdom in nature, a trust that goes beyond any attachment. If we can achieve this greedless state and trust in our higher nature, then we, too, can know the wisdom of trusting the unknown.

Truthfulness

Truthfulness, or satya in Sanskrit, is one of the most important disciplines for the yoga practitioner. For it is through truthfulness that we come to know our eternal Self. Being honest with what we feel, see, and need can be difficult, but it is the basis for trusting our self and others. Surrendering to truth allows us to see things (and ourselves) as they really are, which instills strength of character and a fearlessness to a commitment of honesty that then leads us deeper into integrity.

... If what you are doing in life makes you happy, then ... it is your truth!
—Henry Cory, friend

Integrity is internal honesty. It is telling the truth to yourself and others, even if no one else would know. What would you do if you were standing in line at the grocery checkout and you saw the woman in front of you drop a twenty dollar bill without realizing it? Boy, that extra twenty sure would come in handy for you ... If you picked up the bill and handed it to her, that would be integrity. It could have been so easy to just put it in your own pocket because she didn't even know she dropped it, but because of your moral code of truthfulness, you gave it back to her. Integrity is respecting yourself enough not to deny your truth for any reason.

It's the same concept as you practice yoga. If you deny any of your body's limitations while on the mat, you are potentially causing harm (ahimsa) to yourself. Trying to jump into a handstand without a progressive practice is not only dangerous, it is a denial of your true abilities. In essence, you are lying to yourself and not practicing the truth of your yoga.

Living satya is learning to make conscious choices about telling the truth on your mat and applying it in your daily life. This does not mean telling the truth without diplomacy, for satya (truthfulness) is grounded in ahimsa (non-harming).

Let's say your best friend comes to you for advice on his relationship with his wife and you know that she has not been faithful to him. You would not come right out and say that she has cheated on him and he needs to dump her as fast as he could. That would not be following the moral codes of truthfulness or non-harming, because it would cause him pain for the way you presented the situation. In observing truthfulness, you might ask your friend to go directly to his wife and share with her his concerns about his feelings without bad-mouthing her yourself. If pressed for your knowledge, you might then explain the truth of what you know without interjecting any of your own emotions. Telling the truth in the short term might not always be easy, but it is infinitely valuable in the long run.

Practice: Loving-Kindness

As the Buddha declares in this quote, may *all* beings be at ease. This simple statement of loving-kindness is so completely encompassing that I ask you to try to find any aspect of separateness in its meaning. Loving-kindness is a reflection of integrity basing our actions in compassionate non-harming (ahimsa), which allows us to discover intimacy with ourselves and with others. But, in order to live with integrity, we must be truthful in our lives. Cheating on your college entrance exam and then expecting profound discoveries on your yoga mat is being less than honest with yourself. Using sex as a means of getting your way (rather than for true intimacy) and then expecting to know the essence of unconditional love is outright absurdity. Every aspect of your life is connected, and the sooner you can realize this, the sooner you come to know an awakened life.

May all beings be at ease. Whatever living beings there may be; Whether they are weak or strong, omitting none, the great or the mighty, medium, short or small, the seen and the unseen, those living near and far away, those born and to-be-born—May all beings be at ease!

—The Buddha's words on Loving-Kindness (Metta Sutta)

When we live with personal integrity, we can then feel intimacy for ourselves because we can accept our own actions as truth. In that truth we come to know the inherent goodness within and we fall in love with ourselves. It is this inner love that enables us to love and care for others. Personal intimacy extends outward to all of our relationships and we understand that all beings want to be happy and this helps us to acknowledge our oneness.

Take a few moments now and come into the yoga asana that gives you a sense of well-being. Breathe into it for a few moments, feeling all the bodily sensations. Focusing on your breath, contemplate on all the goodness within yourself. Your mind may want to argue with you and remind you of all those times when you weren't so "good," but tell yourself you are making a commitment to your own happiness and intimacy. Your mind will begin to quiet. As you hold your yoga posture and contemplate your goodness, notice how your body and mind are becoming more integrated.

A Wide-Open Heart

imp. of not being attached

We must release our control over the uncontrollable patterns of life and learn how to connect to love no matter what is happening. Realizing that we cannot hold on to pleasure any more than we can hide from pain will help us flow through our lives in a deeper state of contentment.

Love has no fear. Leap and the net will appear.
—Robert Marinelli, musician

Let's face it, there is no way that we can control growing old and even dying. If we try, we set ourselves up for the mental burdens of hopelessness and disempowerment. But when we consider ourselves as part of a whole, existing in harmony with the cycle of life, feeling connected to our family and friends, and especially to ourselves, we lose the fear of separateness. We jump into life and love with both feet, regardless of a perceived outcome, trusting that we are exactly where we are supposed to be.

The difference between unhappiness and joy depends on where we place our attention. We can choose to transform our thoughts so they embody love and kindness, or we can allow them to get stuck in a habitual loop of believing false concepts of separation.

I remember when I fell in love for the first time. He was a senior and I was a sophomore and I thought he was the most awesome boy in school. There was a spark inside of me that just ignited when he walked into the room and it made me want to spend all of my time with him. Life was good when we were together. Expressing love (or at least intense *like*) and goodwill were easy to do with him.

Then, a month after we professed our undying love for each other, he told me he couldn't see me anymore because he'd fallen in love with someone else. The unexpected news was devastating and I felt rejected and separated from my source of empowerment. What happened to the love? It was still there; however, I chose to place my attention outside of myself on the feelings of rejection. Lucky for me then, being a 15-year-old, I was able to bounce back to those feelings of love when my new boyfriend came into my life a couple of weeks later!

I am not saying that love is shallow and we should not give it its due, but I am suggesting that we, as empowered beings, dig a little deeper into ourselves when the surface happiness and love begin to fade. Find your true source of love inside the wellspring of your heart and let it emanate outward to all those who you come in contact with.

The Compassionate Observer

The words of the Buddha, "life is suffering," makes us want to turn our heads and shy away from the possible thought that life, in fact, is painful. When we see starving children on TV and hear about violence in other countries, or even see the misfortune in the life of our next-door neighbor, we feel overcome by the suffering of another. Sometimes we even think that to be truly compassionate means that we need to be passive and allow others to abuse us. These situations are what we term as having compassion, but it is quite the contrary.

Compassion is strength that arises out of seeing the true nature of suffering in the world. It allows us to witness suffering without fear and to name it. Compassion is having sympathy for all the living without exception and to wish that all beings be free from pain. When we can sense from within ourselves what it must be like to experience someone else's situation, then we have found compassion.

I can still hear the wise words of my mother: "Always be kind because you don't know what that person went through to get here." Likewise, having compassion in your yoga practice can be one of the most profound experiences you will have on and off the mat. Compassion in your practice will expand through your entire life to make your whole existence that of equanimity. Equanimity does not see the world as good and bad or right and wrong, but sees it only as "suffering and the end of suffering." There is no judgment of a situation; fear, guilt, and shame are not a part of your consciousness when you can see life through compassion.

How do we put compassion to work in our yoga practice? When we attempt a pose that is difficult for us and we accept our limitations for that moment, we are acting out of compassion for ourselves. We can see that judgment of our limitation causes suffering but the acceptance of our limitation releases that suffering. This does not mean that we submit to an idea of failure, but that we acknowledge we are in a process of achievement.

When we take this understanding from our mat and apply it to our spouse, children, friends, and co-workers, we can acknowledge their situations with compassion and accept the process of life rather than deny it. To acknowledge the truth of suffering allows us to feel connected with others and to be able to see the truth of life without illusion.

Ustrasana (Camel Pose)

Ustrasana is a very powerful backward bend and demands respect and focus as you perform this posture. It can be one of the most rewarding asanas that you do for the reason of opening your heart and releasing physical and emotional energy that may be stuck in your heart and lungs.

In general, backward bends help to release negative feelings such as depression, lethargy, and dullness of the mind. Ustrasana and backward bends in general are recommended to help relieve depression, although it is wise to seek the help of a professional therapist if your depression is persistent.

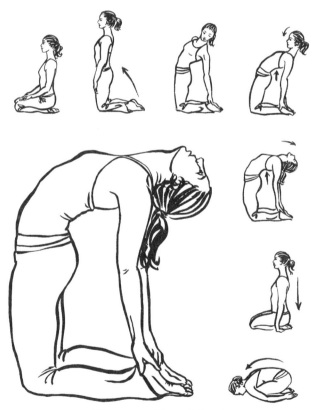

Ustrasana (Camel Pose).

Since this posture stimulates the front side of the body, it affects your power center, which is your solar plexus. This is the place where willpower and inner strength are developed. Stimulation of this area is good for self-confidence.

Empowerment Exercise: Ustrasana

Ustrasana Affirmation: *I am love. My heart is open to all possibilities.*

The underlying feeling with Ustrasana is powerful calm. Try it—ease yourself into this powerfully supportive posture and come to know your self-confident and beautiful spirit!

1. Begin by sitting in Vajrasana (Firm Pose) with your knees bent under your body and your hips resting on your heels. The spine is erect and your arms hang to the sides of your body.

2. Come upright onto your knees and place them about hip width apart, pointing your toes behind you. Let your arms rest at your sides.

3. Tuck your chin toward the chest and inhale deeply. Place the palms of your hands, fingers facing downward, on your hips, press your pelvis forward and lift your chest upward creating an arch in the back.

4. Roll your shoulders back and downward as you release you right hand from your hip and grasp your right heel.

5. Once you have a firm grip with your right hand, reach back with the left hand to grasp onto the left heel. Press the pelvis forward to keep the legs vertical over the hips.

6. Continue lifting upward through your chest, and as you feel comfortable to do so, lower your head back, raising your chin to the sky. (Keep your chin tucked toward the chest if you have neck injuries.)

7. Breathe smoothly as you continue pressing the pelvis forward and lifting the chest, making sure not to sink your weight into the lower back. You may practice this posture for as long as you feel comfortable, but I recommend at least four to eight full rounds of breath.

8. To exit, inhale and bring your chin to your chest, then exhale and pull your body upright and sit back to your heels.

9. Immediately proceed to Balasana (Child Pose) to counter the backward bending motion. Fold forward, resting your forehead on the floor, hips to heels, and resting your arms at your sides, palms facing upward by your feet.

It's important to follow an intense backbend with a forward bend to help even out and balance the energy in the body. Too much backward bending can release large amounts of emotional energy at one time that you may not be ready to handle.

Benefits

Ustrasana stimulates the fourth chakra, your heart center, which affects not only your heart, but also your lungs, sternum, upper back, and even your throat (which is part of your fifth chakra). In breathing into and stretching these parts of your body, you are stimulating prana (life force) and energy to flow through you. This expanding movement encourages fresh, oxygenated blood to flow through your body, which cleanses the organs of your chest. It stimulates your lungs and makes more room for you to breathe.

Most of us have a tendency to hold tension in our upper back, which creates an array of residual neck and shoulder discomfort. Ustrasana increases the flexibility in our upper backs and iliopsoas muscles (hip flexors) which helps to release the tension stored between our shoulders, thus relaxing the backside of our bodies.

Because this posture is such an intense backward bend, it is stretching and lengthening the full front side of your body, thus affecting and stimulating the organs of digestion and reproduction. This pose helps to relieve constipation and is also good to ensure reproductive vitality.

On an energetic level, you can expect emotional releases from minor little feelings of contentment to expansive and overwhelming senses of inner joy, unconditional love, and profound peace. This posture can encourage and release emotions of sadness and grief as well. You may feel anything from a slight moodiness to deep sorrow. Our bodies only release what we store in them. It is wise to befriend and understand your body and the many emotional memories it holds. Ustrasana is one of the most powerful ways we can reach our heart, open it up, release the negative, and accept the joy.

Don't be afraid of what may come up for you. If emotions start to surface, simply breathe into them—deep, full, diaphragmatic breaths—and let them wash away on each exhalation. Notice how your body surrenders into deep relaxation and joy as you complete the posture.

If, for any reason, you feel agitated after doing Ustrasana (or any other backward bend), place your body in a forward bend like Balasana (Child Pose) to help calm the emotional body and soothe the nervous system. It is always best to follow backward bending with forward bends.

Cautions

It is important not to strain as you move into and hold this pose. There are easier variations for you choose from if you feel this posture is too advanced for you. The use of props, such as blocks on either side of your ankles, can help you achieve the benefits of this pose without having to bend into the full extent.

If your neck is weak or has been injured, keep your chin tucked toward your chest throughout the asana. If your neck has been seriously injured, ask your yoga teacher or doctor before you attempt this pose.

Those who have weak or injured knees can place them wider than your hips (8 or 9 inches apart) when moving into this posture. In any case, use extreme caution as you move into this backbend. You may even consider trying a variation or not practicing this asana at all.

If you have cardiovascular diseases such as high blood pressure, history of stroke or heart attack, and/or hardened arteries, try the simpler variations of this pose, and don't hold it for a long period of time. Begin by holding for two full rounds of breath and do not push into the pose. Simply breathe and let your exhalation take you into your extension. An easy variation is to place the heels of your palms on the upper back rim of the pelvis, fingers pointing downward. Tuck your chin toward your chest, press your pelvis forward, and lift your chest and lean into a backbend. The pressure of your hands on the hips helps keep the upper legs vertical and the pelvis tucked.

Do not let fear get in the way of your heart ... remember this with all your friends and with the person you want to love ...
—Henry Cory, friend and fellow "grain of sand"

Real Life

Here is an excerpt from my personal journal. As you can see, my physical practice directly relates to my emotional body and my thoughts. Once again, we are reminded that mind, body, and emotions are all connected to awaken Spirit.

"... I'd been at this retreat for almost two days and I really started to wonder what was wrong with me. I didn't seem to be connecting with anyone, not even myself. The food was awesome, the accommodations were fine, and I'd gotten to do yoga almost all day, every day. For the past few months I had kind of felt detached from my friends and seemed to lose the joy of living, so no wonder I felt disconnected from all the retreat participants ...

... I think I found my problem ... it was my heart.

We did Camel Pose in class today and it felt pretty good so I decided I wanted to do more after class was over, so I found a quiet space and started to lean back into the pose again ... that's when it hit me! My chest started quivering and it took everything I had to stay in the pose and breathe. About that time, Adam (my host and instructor) came up and supported my posture ... he knew what was going on ... so I could breathe better without having to support myself.

As my breathing evened out and got deeper, I began to sob, deep from my gut (try that in a backbend!). I had to come out of the pose and when I did, I just folded into Adam's arms and cried. I cried because I felt joy and I cried because I felt grief. He just let me sob on his shoulder until I couldn't sob anymore. It was a strange mix, but after that experience, I felt so much more love and acceptance for myself as well as everyone around me. I even connected with and made two great friends for the rest of the weekend ... and hopefully longer. I hope this feeling lasts and I know now, how I can bring it back if I ever start to lose it again."

Empowerment Journal

It's time to come back to your empowerment journal. Have you noticed any changes in yourself from your first entry to now? What effect is yoga having on your physical body, but more importantly, what changes have you noticed with your feelings toward yourself, your family and friends, and life in general? Have you noticed a shift in your thoughts from, perhaps, intensity to a more calm and accepting way of viewing your life?

Love bears all things, believes in all things, hopes in all things, endures all things. Love never fails ...
—The Holy Bible, I Corinthians 13:7-8

Take a few moments and add to your journal. These are the memoirs of your empowered Self.

This example from my personal journal captured a particular day when my focus was centered in my heart:

... the sky was a brilliant blue and the sun shined warmly upon my skin, and as I walked to my car after yoga class, I felt strong physically and my head was clear. It was so much easier for me to breathe because my chest felt open. Performing the Wheel was particularly easy for me today and I was delighted, even excited, that I felt so much emotion. I almost cried as I came out of the pose! I even felt pure love and didn't know who to direct it to. I just kept smiling and under my breath said, "Thank you, thank you." Today is a good day to be alive and I just want to hug someone!

Mantras for Daily Living

As I've mentioned, mantras directly affect the vibrations of the chakras by balancing their energy and mantras regarding love and compassion affect the vibrations of our heart chakra. Following are some examples of heart mantras that you can use to help heal a broken heart or just empower your fourth chakra. Feel free to experiment with the mantras in this chapter or make your own, as long as they resonate with you. Remember, a mantra is sacred and resonates with your spirit so it does not have to make total sense to your conscious mind as long as you feel right with your particular recitation.

> Love was born first, the gods cannot reach it, or the spirits, or men ... Far as heaven and earth extend, far as the waters go, high as the fire burns, you are greater, love! The wind cannot reach you, nor the fire, nor the sun, nor the moon: You are greater than them all, love!
> —Atharva Veda 9.2.19

When I begin to feel alone and that love has left my life, I use the mantra, "Love is all there is." Sometimes the music from The Beatles' song "All You Need Is Love" pops into my head and instills my mantra even deeper into my being. This is a good example of turning a mantra into a chant to enforce its healing properties.

Take a few moments now to recite your mantra of love and compassion and then notice how you feel. Physically be aware of your chest and lungs and notice if you feel lighter. Also, pay attention to the change in your mental and emotional states.

- "I give birth to Love in my surrender."
- "Love is all there is."
- "I live with love in my heart and kindness on my lips."
- "Love is the center of my life."
- "Peace, Love, and Compassion."

Giver of the Gifts

Who is the giver and who is the receiver of the gifts in your life? Is it possible that you are both? In following the path of love, we surrender to its unconditional nature. The essence of Real Love knows not the difference between one soul and the next, it acknowledges that we are all One, and in that oneness we open ourselves to the joys and sorrows of our existence.

> Nothing beats the power of Love ... Nothing!
> —Bliss Wood, author and yoga instructor

Through the guidelines of the Yamas, the five moral restraints of non-harming, non-stealing, chastity, non-attachment, and truthfulness, we seek to approach our inner world and outer relationships with integrity through compassion and right action.

Your yoga practice is an invaluable tool for you to come to know your inner Self through body awareness, mental focus, and emotional stability. These qualities, cultivated within you, expand into your daily life to empower your actions of loving-kindness and compassion toward yourself and others. With practice, you will see your life unfold into a state of pure contentment before your very eyes, enabling you to accept the inevitable cycles of suffering as well as the end of suffering until the point you reach your enlightened Self and exist in unconditional love.

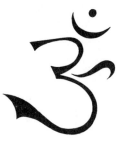

Chapter Five

Finding Strength and Courage

The challenges of life can be daunting. Sometimes we wonder how we will ever make it through the roadblocks and pitfalls we face. Having the right tools to make it through these trouble spots is key to living an empowered life. So what do we do when our world seems to fall down around our feet? It is inevitable that these times arise in our life, but we can meet them head-on with inner strength and courage.

I don't mean to say that we muscle our way through our problems and blindly rush into a situation that we haven't thought through, but that we find a resolve from within ourselves to greet our challenges with the courage of understanding. This is the way of the peaceful warrior who does battle with a pure heart and an open mind. There is no need for the outer combat when the inner awareness is fortified with strength and courage.

The Five Observances (Niyamas)

The niyamas, the second limb, are what Patanjali terms the internal disciplines in the Eight-Limbed Path of the Yoga

Sutras. They address one's personal awareness to the process of realization, whereas the yamas are external disciplines pertaining to how we approach the outside world in which we live.

Through the practices of self-restraint, the niyamas, we create a foundation of awareness and sense of peace with our inner being. We become more of a witness in the actions of our daily life and our mind becomes less reactive and more even-tempered. The ultimate goal in the practice of the niyamas is to deepen our understanding of our true Self. It is through these practices that we come to know grace.

Purity

The first practice of the niyamas is purity or purification. The Sanskrit term is *shauca*. Although this practice refers to bodily cleanliness, its concept reaches further than the mere physical aspect of keeping the body clean and into the deeper sense of inner purification.

> When he has no lust, no hatred, / A man walks safely among the things of lust and hatred.
> —The *Bhagavad-Gita*

According to yoga philosophy (of the Sutras), the ordinary person exists in a state of impurity because of his/her delusions of separateness from God, or the Self. Shauca is the re-awakening of our awareness that we are essentially one with all beings, especially the one true Self. Through the practice of purity, we distance ourselves from our attachments of the body to realize contentment lies within us.

The physical action of keeping our bodies clean is a good foundation for the practice of purity. By eating a proper, healthy diet, getting enough sleep, and bathing regularly, we promote the ability to concentrate, meditate, and let go of outside desires that pull us away from the knowledge of our true Self. However, delving deeper into cleanliness we seek to remove the veil of separation in our minds that keeps us from having a fulfilling relationship with life. When we surrender to that which we find pure (Godliness), we will find the inner strength to support our environment (inner and outer) through our thoughts, words, and actions.

I have a friend who was a major songwriter for a profitable and prestigious publishing company. He was well known in our town and across the country for his number-one hit songs. He had many friends, was quite popular with many of the songwriting organizations, and had amassed some fame and a tidy fortune through his songwriting career, but he wasn't happy. He had been relying on outside kudos and events to bring him peace. He recognized himself as what he was doing rather than who he really was.

It wasn't until he realized that the reason he wasn't happy was because he had shut himself off from his true Self. His Self was not the person who spent his days impressing people with his songwriting talent. Rather, it was someone who desired to know himself on a deeper level.

He eventually quit his job at the publishing company, started his own small business, and began to pursue activities that freed his mind from the extraneous tasks he once mindlessly accepted. Through quite a few years of self-observation and study, he has emerged into a man who no longer needs the approval of someone (or something) else to make him happy. He has found an inner peace with knowing the path to his true Self.

I'm not advocating that we all quit our jobs and hike up into the hills to find enlightenment, but I am suggesting that we begin to ask ourselves these simple questions: "What makes me happy?" and "What is the path of my true Self?"

Your yoga practice can open up the pathway for you to answer these questions and to realize a deeper sense of love, commitment, and understanding not only to yourself, but to God and to family and friends who are extensions of your Self. Taking the time to come to the mat and move into postures that open the heart and steady the mind will begin to clear the way for self-realization. The body-mind connection is powerful and can unlock many truths if you take the time.

Upon rising in the morning, try doing a series of standing forward and backward bends. This will get the blood flowing through your veins, oxygen moving through your lungs, and will also activate your heart center as well as your nervous system. The combination of forward and backward bending will help to balance your body and will stop the chatter of your mind to bring you into present moment awareness where you can begin to know your Self.

Cleanse your life of all the clutter and illusions of separateness and come to know the reality of your pure heart.

Contentment

Can you think of a time when you were truly content in your life, when everything seemed to settle into perfection? Do you remember how it felt to be totally at peace with yourself and the world around you? You felt like you had everything you ever needed and there was no sense of wanting in your mind. Even your body felt relaxed and peaceful.

> That man is happiest who lives from day to day and asks no more, garnering the simple goodness of a life.
> —Euripides, Greek dramatist

Contentment is one of the five moral observances of the Yoga Sutras. Patanjali refers to the Sanskrit word *samtosha*. Its teaching corresponds with the commandment in the Bible of not coveting. When we find peace with what we have and who we are in each moment, we are living with contentment and find that certain things in our life don't really matter. What does count, however, is how we surrender into what is, and how we can accept the inevitable changes that occur in our life. Of course, we can always work toward improvement and at the same time be content in the process. Contentment helps us to know that we are exactly where we are supposed to be in each moment.

These feelings of equanimity come and go throughout our life and we may sometimes feel as if we are on a roller coaster, bumping through the ups and downs of attachment. If we learn to re-evaluate our problems and look at them as opportunities, we can then find contentment as we face our challenges and detach from them. Limitations are nothing more than learning experiences and can be great tools in helping you reach peace and assurance.

Practice contentment on your yoga mat by becoming peaceful with your body and how it moves through the poses. If there is a posture that you have difficulty with, find the serenity to love your body exactly the way it is, perceived flaws and all. Tell your mind that it does not need to explain all your faults. Then take your loving acceptance into your daily life and trust you are exactly where you need to be.

The observance of contentment involves taking responsibility for our lives and the situations in which we find ourselves. It does not mean blaming someone or something else for our problems. Remember, problems are not problems at all, but rather opportunities with which we can achieve greater awareness of ourselves and a better understanding of compassion and acceptance for everything in our life.

One of the most remarkable stories of contentment that I have been so fortunate to personally witness began in July 1995. My mother had been in a near-fatal auto accident while on vacation in the Ozarks and was almost completely immobile when we were able to bring her home to New Mexico. I flew to my parent's home from Phoenix for a couple of weeks to help my father take care of her. Upon my first look at my mom, I had to choke back the tears and breathe through the fear I was experiencing. Once a vibrant, healthy woman, she looked pale and fragile with her numerous casts, cuts, and bruises.

Throughout the time I spent helping her, I experienced every emotion from anger as to why it had to happen to her, to fear of losing my "momma," to gratitude that I still had a mother. I watched her struggle to feed herself, hold a pen, and even sit up in bed. She was in intense pain and yet she was still present with herself and her family. She went from being a mobile, independent woman to someone who needed constant care, and through it all she found contentment in being exactly where she was. She didn't complain but allowed us to help and thanked us for taking care of her. She even remarked that she was grateful for the opportunity to slow down in her life and re-evaluate where she was going.

She was able to admit to herself that she had needed to change directions in her life and hadn't listened until the point of her accident. At that point, she said she stopped worrying about little things like keeping the house clean and watching television, and realized her real happiness came when she spent time with my dad, her children, and grandchildren. She stopped worrying so much and began to smile more. Her regimented ways melted into calmer, more patient acceptance of each present moment. The peaceful, self-assured woman she is today was born in part from her ability to find contentment with what she had in each moment regardless of what had been taken away from her through the accident. She didn't blame anyone, but took responsibility for how she accepted the circumstance.

a problem is not a problem unless you make it one

So it is that we find contentment through patient self-awareness and detachment. There is no freedom sweeter than that of contentment born of taking responsibility for our own life.

Austerity

Tapas, the Sanskrit term for austerity, literally means "heat" or "glow" and refers to the energy that is produced within oneself through discipline and abstinence. Discipline is self-care and must not be confused with denial and self-punishment. Through discipline we create positive energy within ourselves, while self-punishment only serves to destroy our energy. Austerity consists of practices that are meant to test and strengthen our will, not to break it. It promotes our detachment from outside distractions and focuses our mind back to the Self.

Dedicating a specific time each day to your yoga practice is self-discipline. Eating a healthy diet is self-discipline. The concept of "less is more" is a great example of austerity. I don't mean that you should get rid of all your possessions and make do with the bare bones of existence, but in releasing the extraneous trappings of a material world, we gain greater self-control in our lives.

A good friend of mine has taught me the lesson of austerity by the way he lives his life. Although he enjoys material things like many of us, he knows how to live in moderation. His home is clean and sparse, yet he uses everything he owns. Nothing collects dust in closets and there are no piles of "stuff" lying around. He has paid off all of his consumer debt and doesn't allow himself to buy anything he can't afford in the moment. He also has a dedicated yoga and meditation practice which he makes time for every day.

Some people would think that his life is empty and not very exciting, but on the contrary, because he doesn't have extra obligations such as debt and material clutter, he is free to experience life through his choice. Less truly can be more.

Self-Study

Self-study can be a very difficult thing to do if we haven't taken the time to get to know ourselves before now. It is a process of looking deeply into our thoughts, words, habits, and actions. Sometimes we may not like what we see, but it is important to our spiritual growth to shine the light of awareness onto who we really are and what we would like to change.

In Sanskrit, svadhyaya means self-study. This is not the typical studying that we think of, but it is more of a meditative pondering of truth which the heart accesses more so than the mind. Introspection is a better word used to describe the practice of svadhyaya in that it is less of an intellectual learning process and more of a heart-opening practice. When we can look at our life and learn about ourselves through our thoughts and actions, we are in the process of self-study.

For example, I realize that my yoga practice is very important to me; however, at times I tend to deny my own needs for the needs of others and find that I do not always practice as regularly as I should. I allow myself to get distracted with teaching. Mind you, I love teaching yoga, but through my self-study, I realize that I must have balance between being a teacher and being a student. I must allow myself to receive as much as I give. I could not have made this realization through reading a book or taking a test, but the wisdom came when I took time to spend with my own thoughts and actions, evaluating and deciding what is important to me.

In the same way, every time we come to our yoga mat we have the opportunity for syadhyaya. Self-study means paying attention to the physical self. As you center your awareness into your body by breathing into each pose that you attempt, you are able let go of the mind chatter and feel what your body is trying to tell you. How are you holding your body? Are you sitting or standing up straight? Do you feel graceful or clumsy? By asking yourself questions like these, you are actually connecting your mental, physical, and emotional bodies and understanding yourself better.

Self-study also considers how you approach your concept of morality, spirituality, and truth. Do you say what you mean and mean what you say? Do you walk your talk when push comes to shove? If you had to defend your beliefs, would you know exactly what they are? What is your concept of God or Spirit? These are all questions that, when answered, lead to a deeper knowing of Self. Svadhyaya is a tool to help you to realize your true nature.

Devotion

The observance of devotion relates more to matters of the heart than to the intellect. It seeks to open us to the realization that there is a power greater than ourselves. This power is that of our true Self, our God nature.

85

… Cultivating surrender and devotion replaces such self-preoccupation with a sense of our connection that sustains this entire universe.

—Swami Ajaya (Alan Weinstock), author, psychologist, and teacher

This niyama accentuates any form of religion. It is through our devotion to God/our true Self that we relinquish ego and come to live in accordance with our highest potential. Whether your devotion is focused on God, Krishna, Buddha, Great Spirit, or the Universe, your commitment and dedication to your beliefs is the essence of the practice of Ishvar-Pranidhana (devotion).

A sense of devotion and surrender opens us to experiences of being nurtured. When we dedicate time to a yoga practice and surrender to the physical and mental feelings of our work on the mat, we are trusting that we will be supported through our practice. By the same token, worshipping in a church, synagogue, mosque, or outside in nature are all ways in which we show devotion to our God. We learn that we have the capacity to become like God as we commit to a practice of self-awareness through yoga, meditation, and prayer. When we incorporate these practices into our daily lives, we can feel how they enrich our experiences with family and friends, but most of all they enrich the experience we have with our own true Self.

Practice: Prayer

What does prayer mean to you? It has been referred to as "talking to God," while the practice of meditation is "listening to God." For me, prayer is a way of acknowledging my life. When I feel helpless and without answers to my questions, I ask for guidance. When I am overwhelmed with peacefulness, I express my gratitude by smiling and mentally shouting "thank you." Sometimes I'm so grateful for things that I say "thank you" out loud to no one in particular.

I even use my yoga practice as a kind of prayer. As I move from one asana to the next, I focus on the health and strength of my body and give thanks for my abilities. Even if I feel pain as I practice, I concentrate on that pain and ask that it be transformed into healing. Yoga is the best thing I know of for prayer in motion. Once you have established prayer throughout your body while on the mat, it is easy to express that prayer throughout your daily routines.

Think of all the times when you have prayed, whether it was an inter-cession for help, a moment of gratitude, or an acknowledgement of awe and amazement. Do you remember how you felt when you offered those personal and devotional words to God? No matter what you were pray-ing for, you trusted that your words would be heard and your request would be granted. Perhaps you weren't asking for anything, but you felt an overwhelming need to thank the Universe for some gift you received. In either case, they are examples of conversations with your higher Self, or God. They are acknowledgments that you trust a power greater than you to provide for all your needs.

when praying
- guidance
- grateful

Take a few moments and think about what your needs are at this time. Also, think about all the things you have to be grateful for. Make a list of what you want to pray for and then choose two or three yoga postures you can practice while repeating your prayers. For example, you may choose to practice the Warrior Pose and Triangle and a Forward Bend. As you move from one posture to the next, repeat your prayer as you hold each posture. Remember to breathe deeply, instilling your prayers into your body. After about 10 minutes of practice, come to stillness and notice if your heart is at peace and your mind is clear. You may continue this practice for as long as you desire, but make sure you take the time to integrate your mental or verbal prayer with the movement of your body. Trust that you are a living prayer.

The Peaceful Warrior

"Peaceful warrior" somehow seems like a contradiction in terms, doesn't it? *Webster's* dictionary even states in one of its descriptions that peace is "the absence of war." Whether the act of peace is between nations or communities or even peace within the Self, how does being a warrior fit into this relationship?

Peace is liberty in tranquility. ☆
—Cicero, Roman orator and statesman

If we look more closely at the definitions of peace and warrior, we can see more clearly what is meant by the term "peaceful warrior." Peace is a state of serenity or tranquility, while the term "warrior" is explained as a person who has shown great courage. So then, a peaceful warrior is one who with composure and calmness has exhibited fortitude in facing the challenges of life. Courage comes from facing reality. Your strength comes from seeing the obstacle and reaching within for resolve. It is through this looking inward to face your reality that the peaceful warrior exists within you.

In yoga classes, there may be a time when you are challenged to try something that is frightening, either for physical or emotional reasons. The challenge may be a new pose or an adjustment that your teacher thinks you need. Whatever the reason, you must summon your courage to meet the challenge, but how do you do that? One way is to take stock of where you are in the moment. Ask yourself: Am I ready to do this? Do I trust my teacher? Is this situation appropriate for me? Whatever your decision, know that courage is not forcing yourself to do something because someone else thinks it's best for you. Nor is courage doing something for fear you will not be accepted if you decline. We display courage when we find our voice to make our own decisions. If you prefer that your teacher not adjust you, then you would display courage by speaking up and letting her know that an adjustment is not right for you. Any respectful teacher would abide by your wishes and honor them as your truth.

Taking your courage from the mat and into everyday life may feel a little daunting, but you can strengthen your fortitude by acknowledging how many times each day you actually choose to act with courage. The more you recognize these courageous acts, the easier it will be for you to live as a peaceful warrior, making honest choices and standing in your truth.

"Being" Peace

World peace starts with inner peace. Identification with our true nature, which is love, allows us to understand that although nature is continually moving through cycles, our Spirit is completely still. In self-realization we can be peaceful in the midst of chaos. When we can treat everyone (and everything) with kindness, compassion, and unconditional love through our thoughts, words, and actions, we will begin to see peace evolve throughout the world and especially starting in our own life.

He knows peace who has forgotten desire.
—The *Bhagavad-Gita*

Peaceful actions begin with peaceful thoughts. The concept of "thoughts are things" is a most profound teaching in that we regard every mental utterance as having the possibility of affecting our internal and external worlds. Become aware of your self-talk. It is inevitable that our mind speaks to us, and many times it is not as loving as we would like it to be. I can remember the first time I taught a yoga class. I had been practicing yoga for almost 10 years and had been training to be a teacher for some time when the opportunity came for me to teach.

A friend of mine who owned her own yoga studio asked if I would help teach some of her scheduled classes, as she could not take care of the demand on her own. She had every confidence in my abilities and she worked to prepare me for my first class. Even though she was supportive and confident in me, the voice inside my head kept repeating "you're not ready, you're not ready!" It was fear trying to occupy my mind and keep me from moving into the unknown (of teaching). Had I listened to that voice, I might not be the teacher I am today. It is the same with all thoughts we think. If the thought is a violent or unhealthy thought, then that is what we are asking the Universe to provide us. If our thoughts are positive, loving thoughts, that is what we bring to us.

"Being" peace requires that we take responsibility for our thoughts as well as our actions. It is an understanding that we are connected to all beings and thus are required to think and act with their, as well as our, well-being in mind.

we are a part of sthlarger

Have you noticed how other people's moods affect you? Perhaps you've even known what someone else was going to say before they even said it. These are examples that show us how connected we are to others. Imagine what our world would be like if we all took the time to "be" peace.

Virabhadrasana (Warrior Pose)

When you think of a warrior, do you visualize sword-slinging, armor-wearing soldiers who defend their homelands in battle? The yogic warrior, however, is one who can balance in the midst of chaos, staying calm and clearheaded, able to meet his or her challenges with courage and inner strength. This warrior is one who takes the time to understand the situation she is in and calmly and gracefully takes action.

The key to working through your resistance is always a radical inner surrender, a calm determination, and a commitment to letting go!
—Baron Baptiste, yoga instructor and author

When attempting to hold the Warrior Pose, most of us will automatically tense up in preparation for "battle" at the mere utterance of the word. The term "warrior" tends to conjure up images of strife and fighting, but if you come to the Warrior Pose with the thought of calm, inner strength, you can easily surrender your body to a firm, yet supple pose. Approach the Warrior with self-assuredness and you will know its true representation of an open mind and the expansion of consciousness.

One of my students in California who owned her own accounting business was a very hard worker and a good boss. She was fair and friendly to her clients as well as her staff, but she kept having the sense that she was going in circles. Her life seemed like a constant battle to keep up with her work as well as find the quality time to spend with her husband. She told me she thought the harder she worked, the farther behind she fell.

When she finally asked if I would teach yoga to her company for stress reduction, her doctor had told her that she needed to "de-stress or else." Her most important reason for starting yoga was to enjoy living again.

She and I worked together one-on-one at first before shifting into a class setting. As she told me about her life, I began to realize that what she needed was more internal stamina to help focus her external activities. We began with a session of Ujjayi Breath (discussed in Chapter 7), some hip openers to help ground her, and then intermittent periods of the Warrior Pose to increase stamina and courage.

In the beginning of our sessions, it was difficult for her to stay in the Warrior Pose very long. She became fatigued and her muscles would shake. It was hard for her to keep her eyes focused down her extended arms. Eventually, as she incorporated Ujjayi Breath into Virabhadrasana, she began to stand for longer periods of time with her arms extended. Her breath was deeper and more even, and her gaze became soft yet steady and focused.

By the time we shifted our practice to a classroom setting, she not only was standing in Warrior Pose with a supple yet strong stance, she had managed to organize her office in such a way that she had time for her personal life as well as finding *new* clients. Not only was her personal life on track, but her business was now growing instead of stagnating!

You may be asking yourself if yoga is powerful enough to change someone's outside world so dramatically. In seeing (and feeling) for yourself, you will come to understand the dramatic changes occur on the inside first through discipline, courage, and inner strength, and then expand outwardly. Your daily life is a reflection of your internal strength, your warrior.

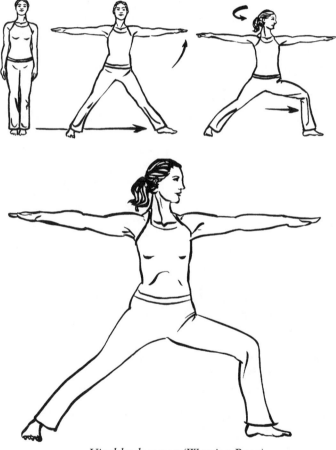

Virabhadrasana (Warrior Pose).

Empowerment Exercise: Virabhadrasana

Virabhadrasana Affirmation: *Through my inner strength I have the willpower to live my life with courage.*

A grounded, wide stance is characteristic of this asana. Your arms are extended straight out from your body as you calmly gaze over your shoulder, bringing your focus back to your core. As you lift up your torso, straightening the spine and grounding deeper into your legs, notice how tension begins to melt away and your legs create a solid foundation. Concentration fills your mind the more you are able to surrender into your own strength. It's easy to take your newly found focus and apply it to the situations of your life.

1. Begin in Tadasana (Mountain Pose, see Chapter 1) and step your feet apart about 3 or 4 feet. Turn your left foot out 90 degrees and turn your right foot inward about 20 degrees. Make sure that your left knee points in the same direction as your left foot. (Although it is best to face your pelvis forward, it is more important to align the foot and knee.)

2. Inhale and raise your arms out to the side, shoulder height, keeping the palms facing downward as you lift your chest and roll your shoulders down your back. Exhale.

3. Inhale once again and elongate your spine upward, then exhale and bend your left knee directly over your ankle into a sideways lunge. Your chest is still facing forward. Keep your hips level and your torso straight, making sure your shoulders are relaxed, down away from your ears.

4. Once you have come into the lunge, without shifting your torso, turn your head only to the left, gently gazing over your left fingers. Keep your chin parallel to the floor.

5. Breathe evenly and naturally as you hold the pose. Remember to relax your jaw and shoulders as you continue to lengthen up through your spine.

6. To release from this pose, inhale and press your left foot into the floor, straightening your left knee, and rotate your head back to your center. Exhale.

7. Turn your feet parallel to each other, keeping a lift in your chest as you lower your arms back to your sides.

8. Step back into Mountain Pose and breathe, integrating the effects of Warrior Pose.

9. Repeat to the right side.

Benefits

There are many benefits to practicing the Warrior Pose. On a physical level, this posture strengthens the legs, especially the quadriceps. It helps to increase your physical groundedness. It also improves your posture and invigorates the spine.

Mentally, through the increased amount of oxygen flowing through the body, it allows you to focus your thoughts and release distractions. Generally, it is very stimulating; however, you will find it to have a calming affect on the mind.

This pose also strengthens your first and third chakras (see Chapter 1). It has the ability to support our self-confidence, which radiates from our solar plexus (our power center) by engaging the stomach muscles throughout the pose. A strong, supported leg stance also supports the first chakra, which is associated with foundation.

Ultimately, Virabhadrasana develops a sense of courage, inner strength, groundedness, willpower, and calmness. Come to this posture whenever you feel that your internal power is low or you are feeling out of balance with life.

Cautions

There are a few things to consider when doing the Warrior Pose. It is important to keep your bent knee directly over the ankle and not over-flex. Your posture is the most solid and supported when the knee is over the ankle. As the knee extends past the ankle and foot, you begin to lose your center and solid base.

It is also important to keep your hips relaxed, even though your legs are your point of strength in this pose. Do not force the pelvis open; let it open naturally. As you continue to practice, you will notice that an open pelvic girdle comes more readily.

Especially if you are pregnant and have a tendency toward swayback, be mindful to tuck your pelvis and draw your navel in toward the spine. It is a good reminder for all who practice Virabhadrasana to be mindful of your lower back.

Real Life

Here is a fun real-life story from Desiré. She and I met about two years ago when we helped to open a healing arts center for the community in Nashville, Tennessee. I could see she had an adventurous spirit with lots to offer the new program.

"Wonder Woman was my favorite role model growing up because her courage and confidence were so appealing, and I always longed for that kind of inner strength.

One day in yoga class, after an especially emotional week, I found myself very fatigued in Warrior Pose. It would have been so easy for me to give up at that moment. As my muscles shook and my concentration grew, I realized that both strength and surrender are a necessary part of every yoga pose and this gave me the courage to continue standing in this posture. This paradox allowed me to accept my limitations and appreciate my practice in brand new ways.

I've lost over 75 pounds doing yoga ... so yoga has become my new best friend! My appetite has changed to crave healthier foods, I'm now thirsty for water instead of sugary drinks, I sleep more soundly and wake up more energized, my sinuses have cleared up, and even my eyesight has improved. I'm so grateful for the time I spend doing yoga, mostly because every session brings me closer to my Wonder Woman warrior within."

Empowerment Journal

Your empowerment journal doesn't always have to reflect a certain pose or an emotional feeling, but can encompass philosophical realizations and insights as to how yoga has touched your entire life. Give yourself free rein to write of your experiences with yoga, whether you discuss a certain event or feeling or perhaps you may want to generalize a thought.

Here is an excerpt from an essay that William, one of my students, wrote regarding his experience of yoga. Even though he does not discuss one particular pose, he embodies the essence of yoga through his experiences on and off the mat:

How has yoga affected my life? I attempt to live everything in relation to a God that I do not know but believe in blindly. Yoga enables me to pursue that endeavor not only on the spiritual plane but also in the body, deep into the inaccessible recesses of my limbs and internal organs. It bathes them in energies released from within and exchanged with the surrounding world. It gives me a feeling of relative control over my life from its physical grounding on up. Pain seems a little less ineluctable than it did before. My body is not condemned to just suffer fatalistically, but can seek out its weaknesses and vulnerabilities, confront them, and work with them. I can do this at a pace of my choosing, gauged so that I can stand it and even enjoy it, rather than waiting to be wracked and helpless. I can even step out ahead of the inevitable accumulation of problems and cultivate the vibrancy that wards off evil. The reassurance this practice gives me inspires gratefulness and issues in praise. Yoga has become a form of prayer for me, an integral part of my prayer life.

yoga as a modern form of prayer

Mantras for Daily Living

Take a few moments now to choose your mantra of courage, inner strength, and willpower. Once you find one that resonates deeply with you, recite it out loud for at least a minute then notice how you feel. Physically, be aware of your abdomen (solar plexus) and your legs. Notice if you feel any sensations of heat welling up in your belly. Perhaps you are feeling a combination of solid strength and at the same time relaxation in your legs and feet. This feeling is groundedness.

Also, pay attention to the change in your mental and emotional states. Are you beginning to feel calm? Is your mind starting to have a pinpointed focus? Make sure you are focused without having tension in your eyes or shoulders, but mostly release the tension of your thoughts.

Become aware of your emotions and see if you are experiencing more confidence and courage, and a calm inner strength. Let the Warrior Pose bring you to that calm yet solid place deep within you. Find your empowered Self!

- "I am greater than all my challenges."
- "I release fear by believing in myself."
- "My courage empowers me with inner strength."

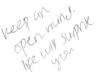
keep an open mind. life will surprise you

- "I stand grounded in my truth and open to new possibilities."
- "I am confident in my ability to make life work."
- "I choose the power of life."

if there's a will there's a way

How Do You Fit in Your Own Life?

Between your job, running the kids to dance lessons and ball practice, fixing dinners, volunteering at your church, and being available for your spouse, if you have one, where do you fit into your life? Do you find that more times than not, there isn't enough time during the day to take care of yourself? This may sound crazy, but those of the Eastern philosophy look upon the "busyness" of the West and refer to us as being lazy! Because we clutter our lives with tasks and to-do lists, and don't take time to process what it is we are actually doing, we ignore the very essence of who we are and why we're here. In other words, we are spiritually lazy, afraid to look deeper into our true Self as we hide behind the never-ending activities in our lives.

diff. but phys. + spirit (wellness)

⊛ key concept

Wherever you live is your temple, if you treat it like one.
—The Buddha

It's important to remember that we have the power of choice. Life does not just happen to us. It's true that things happen that are out of our control, but we have the ability to make a choice in how we deal with the situations that are given to us.

Start right now to fit back into your life. Make the commitment to a yoga or meditation practice and figure out what you really want. Find contentment with your daily activities and release those events and activities that no longer serve you. Through self-awareness and dedication to living in peace, you will not only fit into your life, but it will become a transformational experience full of joy, love, and greater awareness.

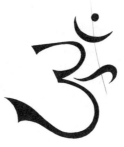

Chapter Six

Stretching Beyond Limiting Beliefs

It isn't always easy reaching out of complacency and into the unknown, but if we are to evolve to a higher consciousness, then we have to stretch beyond the perceived boundaries we have made for ourselves. If something isn't working for you anymore, it is perfectly fine to find a better way of achieving your goals. Just because your best friend always eats fish on Fridays because it is a religious preference doesn't mean you have to do the same thing, especially if you don't like fish! There are many ways to honor your spirit and your beliefs without limiting them. Honor your friend for her dedication and then find your own special, unique way of experiencing your life.

Ours is a society of fast cars, fast food, urgent phone calls, and last-minute meetings. The list could go on forever, but you get the idea! With all this rushing around we tend to put our senses on autopilot. When our minds get so overloaded with "busyness," we begin to shut down our creative thinking process and become like zombies, which in turn keeps us stuck in limited belief systems. It is much easier to "follow the crowd" than to break away into our own curiosity when we are overworked and don't take time for stillness.

If we are to realize our true Self and break away from the limiting structures and beliefs that don't serve us anymore, then we must make room for new ideas and experiences that will support an empowered life. We must bring our awareness back to that centered place of stillness within our body and mind. It is through this focused stillness that we reach beyond our stagnant beliefs and come to experience unlimited possibilities.

Hatha Yoga

Hatha Yoga is the physical practice of yoga. Hatha is esoterically translated to mean union between the sun and moon which ultimately describes the joining of two great forces, the body and mind ("Ha" describes sun and "tha" describes moon). It is the third limb of Patanjali's Yoga Sutras. The ultimate purpose of the physical aspect of yoga is to bring enlightenment in the present moment to a transcended immortal body. In other words, yoga postures are meant to bring our body/mind connection into a state of balance and harmony.

> Glorify God in your body.
> —The Holy Bible, I Corinthians 20

Hatha Yoga plays a very important role in helping us to "wake up" to our full potential to give, to receive, to love, to feel, to achieve total body/mind/spirit awareness. The most important benefit in this practice is not so much the flexibility and the ability to stand on your head, but awareness. The goal of yoga is as much being mindful on your mat as it is in participating in life to the fullest extent. Feelings of integration develop as we begin to sense a deeper connection between our mat practice and our daily tasks.

I have many students who have commented on how the perceptions of their lives changed after practicing yoga even for as short amount of time as one month. One student told me he quit drinking socially because it didn't feel necessary to him anymore. Another student said that he used to have terrible road rage but it disappeared after he started his yoga practice. One woman explained that yoga helped her to see her children in a different way. Rather than being irritated by their naturally childish ways, she was able to delight in the fact that they were happy and healthy and enjoying their childhood. She felt grateful for having her kids, whereas she once felt trapped and frustrated. So you see, we do yoga for more than just the physical results. We do it to enrich our daily lives and to have greater access to our spirit.

Asanas

Our posture is one of the most basic and overlooked aspects of good health and a happy life. Because we have been taught to deny the body, it stands to reason why we don't consider our posture. In the practice of Hatha Yoga, each asana is to be experienced only as long as we are comfortable holding it. Asanas are created situations of stress in which we learn to integrate our body, mind, and breath to work through areas of fear, rigidity, and self-imposed limitations. As our body becomes more flexible, so does our mind. We begin to release our preconceived attitudes about the way life "should" be, and accept each moment as it is. Instead of feeling the urge to change once painful and limiting situations, we simply change our attitudes about them, which in turn releases our attachment to control and reduces stress.

body + mind flexibility

> The human shape is a ghost made of distraction and pain. Sometimes pure light, sometimes cruel, trying wildly to open this image tightly held within itself.
> —Rumi, poet

Asana is the Sanskrit word for posture or pose; however, its deeper meaning stems from the Sanskrit root word "Stah" which means to establish steadiness and firmness. Translated to mean "seat" or "place," asana then is a form of steadiness that leads to deep inner stillness.

steadiness = stillness

You may have noticed that all the names of the yoga poses in Sanskrit have "asana" on the end of the word. In the following table are some examples of the Sanskrit terms with the root word meanings, pronunciation, and the English translation. The poses listed here are explained in more detail throughout this book.

Name of Pose, Translation, and Pronunciation	Described in Chapter
Tadasana (Mountain Pose) tada = mountain tah-dah'-sah-nah	1
Ardha Matsyendrasana (Half Spinal Twist) matsyendra = lord of the fish ahr'-dhah maht-syen-drah'-sah-nah ardha = half	3
Ustrasana (Camel Pose) ustra = camel oos-trah'-sah-nah	4
Virabhadrasana (Warrior Pose) vira = hero bhadra = kind, gracious, happy, blessed veer-ah-bah-drah'-sah-nah	5
Trikonasana (Triangle Pose) tri = three know = angle tree-koh-nah'-sah-nah	6
Parvatasana (Seated Mountain Pose) parvata = seated mountain pahr-vah-tah'-sah-nah	8
Natarajasana (Dancing Shiva Pose) nata = actor, dancer, mime raja = king not-ah-raj-ah'-sah-nah	9
Siddhasana (Perfect Pose) siddha = perfected being seed-hah'-sah-nah	10
Padmasana (Lotus Pose) padma = lotus pod-mah'-sah-nah	10
Savasana (Corpse Pose) sava = corpse shah-vah'-sah-nah	11
Sirsasana (Headstand Pose) sirsha = head sir-sah'-sah-nah	12

Physical Effects

In all asana sequences, it is wise and suggested to use counter poses to take our bodies in the opposite direction from the previous pose or series of poses. Counter poses help balance our body and eliminate any resistance and/or strain that may accumulate in our practice. For example, after completing a forward bend such as Adho Mukha Svanasana (Downward Facing Dog), it is wise to follow that pose with a backward bend such as Urdhva Mukha Svanasana (Upward Facing Dog). The forward bend soothes the nervous system while the backward bending movement stimulates your emotional body.

A well-rounded practice consists of a combination of forward and backward bends, twists, balancing poses, inversions, standing, and seated as well as relaxation postures. While some styles of yoga have a consistent postural routine, others do not, and the practice can change daily. Both approaches are good. The key is to find the practice that best fits your body and lifestyle.

Following is a list of the types of poses you might experience in your yoga practice. A combination of these bends, twists, and stretches are most beneficial to a well-rounded practice:

- Forward bends induce an experience of deep peace and serenity. They also balance the effects of backward bends.

- Backward bends are perhaps the most useful asanas for energizing the body. The movement of the back-bending pose lends itself to opening the heart and therefore helps to stimulate the emotional body to bring balance to our moods.

- Spinal twists are cooling and rejuvenating and are great to help relieve tight back muscles and stress from spinal nerves. They are particularly good to do after a strenuous yoga routine.

- Inversions are important for their ability to bring energy and life force (prana) to the brain. The definition of an inverted pose is one in which the heart is lower than the abdominal organs. Standing Forward Bend (Uttanasana) as well as Headstand (Sirshasana) are both considered inversions. Backward-bending motions are good counter poses for inversions.

- Standing poses help to create stability and strength in the body and mind. There are many balancing postures that are part of the standing asanas. They promote centeredness and focused, energetic action and are a good counter to the seated poses.

- Seated postures promote stillness in mind and body while they also prepare us for meditation. It is good to follow standing postures with seated or relaxation poses to balance the energetic outward energy with internal stillness.

It is important to give our bodies the time to absorb the experiences of our practice as we bring attention back to the Self. Therefore, taking time to integrate the feelings in between each asana is imperative to help us instill our yoga practice in our very cells. When our yoga lives in our cells, it lives in us and our lives are changed forever.

Beyond the Body

Proper alignment is just the beginning of our yoga practice. The deeper awareness we experience through yoga has to do with tuning into and directing the energy flow of each pose. This requires coming into a state of stillness and inner awareness, even as our body holds a posture that may be challenging. This is one reason why a regular meditation practice is vital to experiencing a deeper level of Hatha Yoga.

> The body is mortal. It is subject to death. Yet it is the resting place of the immortal, incorporeal Self.
> —*Chandogya Upanishad*, ancient yogic text

Meditation and yoga are synergistic in that they complement each other for the practitioner to achieve enlightenment. Stilling the mind through meditation enables us to relax more fully into yoga. At the same time, our physical practice of asana relieves our body from the pain and stress it holds so as to calm the mind and help it to release vritti (scattered thoughts) and focus on God-realization.

So many of my students and fellow yoga practitioners have stated how much the physical practice of yoga has influenced their daily decisions, changed their outlooks on life, and even brought about life-changing events such as the ability to quit smoking, become vegetarian, and even make major career changes. This is not to say that we ignore our bodies or consider them less than our Spirit, but we put into perspective that we are all and more than our bodies. When we live from a clear mind, an open heart, and a healthy body, we are truly living life beyond the body. We are experiencing the Self.

Practice: Empowered Movement

How do you define empowered movement? There are no wrong answers because empowered movement can mean many different things to different people. For me, empowered movement is taking action in a conscious and clear way, whether it means I donate to a local charity, practice deep breathing exercises, or perfect my Triangle Pose on the mat. As long as I am acting in a way that makes me feel strong yet compassionate, wise yet humble, then I am expressing empowered movement.

Try this experiment and see how it makes you feel. Think of some task that you have been putting off because you're either not sure of how to do it or you already know that it's not such a pleasant experience. This could be paying bills, renewing your driver's license at the DMV, making a doctor's appointment, or repairing that leaky faucet in the bathroom. Whatever it is, make the choice right now to complete the task. Give yourself a deadline (the sooner the better so you don't procrastinate on that too!) and "just do it!"

If you need moral support, go to your yoga mat and practice Triangle Pose (explained later in this chapter) and Warrior Pose (see Chapter 5), and follow them with Mountain Pose (see Chapter 1) to integrate the feelings of strength, courage, and surrender. Notice how much easier it is to complete the task after you have moved your body and mind through these asanas.

Playing Your Edge

Strive to challenge your body by playing your edge. Experience your own limitations and then breathe through them. As you realize your physical limitations, breathe into the tightness and as you exhale, feel your body surrender and relax, able to move past your original limitation.

No one knows what he can do until he tries.
—Publilius Syrus, Latin writer of mimes (first century B.C.)

Our breath is the most important tool we have to help us experience yoga postures in a deep, surrendering way. If we direct our inhalation to the areas where we feel tension, and then surrender into our exhalation, we can feel our bodies relax deeper into each pose. Our muscles will begin to soften, which will allow us to shift into relaxation.

It takes time to move into the full extent of a pose, so don't forcefully push yourself to your edge in the first breath. Inhale and feel your breath move into the places of tightness. Let it expand fully, creating space for your body to move deeper into the pose on your exhale. Feel yourself relaxing as you exhale, surrendering into the essence of the asana.

It is important to remember that if we strain and push our body's edge we create a block in our energy instead of opening up to it. This can cause us to feel more tension in the body as well as in the mind. If you are practicing an asana such as Triangle Pose, and you feel frustration or agitation, check with your body to see if you are holding tightness anywhere. Are your hips relaxed? Is your neck elongated and aligned with your spine? Are you breathing deeply? Generally, if your mind is preoccupied and agitated, it is reflecting tension in the body. Let your body move with the flow of your breath and notice how your mind and body surrender to the movement and benefits of each posture you attempt.

Take a Stand

We need a balance of awareness not only between the mind and body, but also between security and freedom. It is important for us as self-actualized beings to experience the freedom of our imaginations and our creativity through our bodies. At the same time, in our human experience, we feel a need for security to assure us that who we are and what we are doing is right. Ultimately, though, it is impossible to have freedom if we cling to security at all costs. If we are so busy holding on to our security blankets (such as money, titles, people, or images), there is no room in our consciousness for creativity and the freedom to explore the unknown.

Everything possible to be believed is an image of truth.
—William Blake, English poet and mystic

It's time to take a stand in our lives and experience security through the risks we take. Start by breathing a little more deeply into your yoga postures and be more active in playing your edge. Become more willing to explore and take responsibility for the emotions and thoughts that come up for you during yoga class. Be honest with yourself in your practice and then begin to see how it applies to your life.

Through acknowledging yourself, your limitations and strengths on the mat, you realize that you come to your yoga with some hesitancy yet with an open heart. How does this relate to your real life? Perhaps the hesitancy stems from questioning your abilities as a parent or a lover. Maybe your self-confidence has been shaken because you've been laid off from your job. Deep inside you are excited to start your own business now that you have the time and freedom to do so. This feeling comes from having an open heart.

Whatever the circumstances are in your life, you can bet they will reflect in your yoga practice. By the same token, your practice will afford you the stillness and clarity to come to terms with your life situations.

Standing poses are excellent in giving us the courage to "take a stand" in our lives. They give us a simultaneous feeling of stability and expansiveness, one blending into the other. However, they require great internal focus and commitment. Think of the focus it takes to ground yourself into the Triangle Pose and still lift upward through your chest and arm. This is not a simple relaxing posture and requires a commitment to an open heart, expanded mind, and a solid, supportive body.

Feel the benefits of standing poses—stability, strength, courage, expansiveness, and creativity—and see how life-changing and empowering they can be in your day-to-day experiences.

Trikonasana (Triangle Pose)

Trikonasana is an active standing posture that can breathe life and energy into your whole being. It is a combination of a standing and balancing pose. This translates into an asana that instills a grounded foundation (through standing) and a sharp yet calm internal mental and physical focus (through balancing). Whenever you are feeling that you have lost your power, your internal fire, and your zest for life, or if you can't seem to focus on the task at hand, try spending some time breathing in Triangle Pose. When you are feeling stagnant and stuck in old ways of thinking or your life and relationships feel boring and uneventful, try practicing Trikonasana and feel how it energizes your body and changes your outlook on life. It will clear your head, focus your mind, and energize your body. It can also do wonders to help boost your self-confidence.

The angles of Trikonasana are very pronounced. If you observe the posture, you will notice the arms create a perpendicular line while the torso creates a horizontal line in the body. The straddled legs, which are your foundation, form diagonal lines, thus creating the triangle shape. The following illustrations show the lines of Triangle Pose.

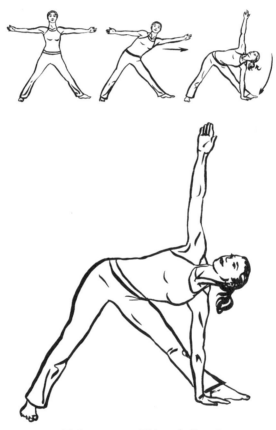

Trikonasana (Triangle Pose).

Empowerment Exercise: Trikonasana

Trikonasana Affirmation: *As I connect to the earth, I reach to my highest potential!*

A triangle has a solid base and lifts up into one focal point. So it is with your body as you practice this pose. Your legs create a solid base as your body extends and your arms reach to that one pointed focus. There is no denying the power and strength that is instilled in you when you practice Triangle Pose!

1. Begin in Tadasana (Mountain Pose, see Chapter 1) and step your feet about three to four feet to the sides.

2. Turn your right foot out 90 degrees and turn your left foot in about 20 degrees. Make sure that your left knee directly points over the foot.

3. Inhale and raise your arms out to your sides at shoulder height, palms facing forward. Roll your shoulders down your back as you extend through your arms. Exhale.

4. Inhale and extend up through your spine, lifting from the crown of your head and keeping your tailbone dropped toward the floor. Exhale.

5. Inhale and reach your left arm and torso to the left as you release your left hip downward. Make sure your spine is straight from your tailbone through your neck and your left rib cage long and open.

6. As you exhale, lower your left arm toward your leg and place your left hand on that leg (avoiding your knee). You may place your hand to the floor if your body can comfortably extend that far.

7. Raise your right arm to the sky, keeping both arms in a straight vertical line. Turn your head to look up toward the right hand.

8. Breathe deeply and stabilize into this position. Roll your right hip (the top hip) back to help open the front of your body.

9. Extend through your legs and keep them straight and strong. At the same time, continue extending your arms in opposite directions as you elongate through your spine.

10. To exit this pose, inhale, tuck in your stomach to support your lower back, and turn your head to face forward. Exhale. Press into your legs and lift from your right arm straight up, feeling as if someone were pulling you up by your right hand.

11. Exhale, step your feet together, back into your Mountain Pose and breathe deeply to integrate the feelings of this posture.

12. Repeat to the right side.

Benefits

Trikonasana is an excellent way to expand your chest, improve balance, and support a strong healthy back. It actively stretches and elongates the spine while opening the chest to allow greater lung capacity. This standing posture provides a dynamic experience of balance in the body and centered focus in the mind.

Triangle Pose stretches and strengthens the hamstring and lateral muscles around the spine. This can help relieve lower back pain by releasing the lower three chakras and allowing prana (life force) to flow through your solar plexus, sacral region, down through the tailbone, and into your legs and feet. This is a powerful, grounding pose.

Another wonderful benefit of Trikonasana is the stimulation of the kidneys and adrenal glands, which promotes a healthier urinary tract and endocrine system. Because of the extension and twisting motions through the torso, it is also beneficial for the organs of assimilation, such as the small and large intestines.

Even though this is considered a standing posture, Trikonasana has great benefits to your ability to balance. As you continue practicing this pose you will feel a sense of grace as well as strength moving through your entire body. The ways you can bring this grace to your daily life is through your ability to express yourself. Trikonasana supports your third chakra, the solar plexus, which is the area of self-confidence and personal strength (see Chapter 1). Your belly is your power center and Trikonasana will support you as you stand up for yourself and present your gifts to the world.

Cautions

As powerful and positive as Trikonasana is, there are a few cautions to consider in order to maintain optimal health in your joints and muscles. As with everything we do in life, moderation and consideration are the keys.

If you have weak or injured knees, it is wise to approach this posture with caution. Do not spread your feet too wide as this causes more strain on weakened knees. Be mindful of your leading knee (the one you are leaning toward) and bend it if necessary to take pressure off the joint. Take your time descending into the posture and don't lean over as far to begin with.

Take your time moving into this strong pose and pay attention to what your body is telling you. If you listen to your body and breathe deeply, you will achieve the benefits of this asana without injury.

Real Life

I met Susan about three years ago while I was teaching yoga at a local health club in Nashville. She was witty and sometimes reverently irreverent in class, displaying a playful yet dedicated approach to yoga. Her enthusiasm was contagious and her love for yoga apparent. This real-life experience from her takes us on a journey of self-discovery from the mat to the contemplations and realizations of her life.

"My yoga journey began many years ago in New York, where I grew up. Upon entering my first yoga class, I knew I was home. The practice seemed to fit so well with my life and it has lived in my heart ever since.

I have been practicing yoga for a few years now and have been introduced to several different asanas. What I have learned is that all the poses, much like people, are connected and intertwined. Each pose seems to lend itself to the next and I can see and feel how they affect my body and my mind. Waves of the ocean ebbing and flowing with the tides reminds me of how each posture flows into the other.

The Triangle Pose is perhaps one of my favorite postures in Hatha Yoga. At first glance it appears extremely difficult in nature. I was instantly reminded of the childhood game Twister where the participants stretch and reach across each other to find their places ... left foot red ... right foot yellow ..., and so forth. I thought that I would virtually have to become Gumby in order to do this pose.

I am so grateful, however, for the wonderful instructors that I have had over the years. I was told just to listen to my body and go only as far as it would allow and to close my eyes and lead with my heart, not my mind. This has helped me to tune out all the negative thoughts that flood my mind during yoga practices. With the guidance of my instructors and my own willingness to achieve the Triangle, my body gave way and I was able to let go and let it fall into the position it was able to move into.

I was once told that life happens in moments and that the hardest thing to do is to be present in those moments. Trikonasana has helped me to become present in the moments of my life. The essence of this asana is strength, balance, and surrender.

The strength part of this pose is coming slowly as I learn to develop a conscious awareness of my body and muscles and how they all work together.

Balance is also a real key to this pose for me. It is something I still have to struggle with in my own life on a daily basis. It's a virtue that I have learned to create for myself. It is essential not only in this pose and for many other poses in yoga, but it is essential in my life as a whole.

Surrender, which is the last key element of this posture, was the hardest for me to grasp. Ever since I was a child I fought surrendering. To surrender, I thought, was to give up, to quit, to lose. I was not going to admit powerlessness. Yet through my yoga practices I have learned that surrender is a positive thing. When I truly surrender and am humble on the mat as well as in life, that is when real growth begins. Surrender is key in the Triangle Pose for me. The deeper I can surrender into the pose, the further my body can move into the posture without resistance.

I take the lessons and elements of the Triangle Pose and implement them throughout my life. I am learning to be strong and balanced. I am learning to surrender in order to grow and receive in my life.

The asanas of my yoga practice today are not only poses, but they are life lessons. My willingness to be open to the lessons provides the key to my growth not only in my practice, but throughout my entire life. I am grateful for the awareness that my yoga practice has granted me and I am continually blessed by its wisdom."

Empowerment Journal

Once again, it's time to take a look at your empowerment journal. Have you noticed any changes in your practice since you have been keeping records of your feelings, whether they were physical, emotional, or both? Perhaps you have discovered that your mental state is more positive and proactive, rather than depressed and stagnant.

Even if you do not have a formal journal to write in, just the act of writing down your thoughts and feelings after doing a yoga posture can help you become aware of what your body is trying to tell you.

I try to write in my journal every chance I get. It helps me to sort my feelings and thoughts, and especially, it helps me to make sense of why I do yoga and how it supports my full life. Here is another sample of my thoughts as I contemplate Trikonasana:

The Triangle posture has become one of my favorite poses in that when I practice it, I can feel my whole body respond. Without feeling my ego, I still feel a sense of self-confidence wash over me, which gives me mental focus and a quiet heart. For some reason I truly understand what it means to feel empowered when I do this pose. It's hard to explain, but unlike some of the other postures, I can immediately find strength as I reach over to each side and extend my arms vertically.

My body moves in stages with this pose. First, I feel my sides elongate as I reach and lean over, then my legs feel their strength as they hold me up. The most exciting part of this pose to me is the ability to completely relax my hips and then feel a deep twist through my spine. At that point, I can lift my chest, draw my shoulders down my back, and feel like I am floating ... awesome!

Mantras for Daily Living

By now, chanting a mantra may be becoming second nature to you. Have you noticed how much more powerful your yoga practice is when you recite your mantra as you move into each asana?

If you haven't yet used your mantra while doing yoga, can you think of a time during your day when you found yourself repeating a certain word or phrase? Perhaps a song lyric kept repeating in your head. Can you remember how that recitation seemed to fuel you through whatever it was you were doing?

Here's a childhood story about the little choo-choo train who "knew he could." I remember this story like it was yesterday. In a very abbreviated version, this little train chugged along, doing his job with pride. As he began to cross the steep mountain he began to chug out loud, "I think I can, I think I can, I think I can ..." until he came to the other side of the mountain and said "I know I can."

The moral of this simple childhood tale is to believe in ourselves. The yogic lesson is that through the power of spoken word, mantra, we live our intentions and achieve our goals. We must never underestimate the power of sound and its ability to heal us.

Here are some suggestions for your mantra choice that relate to letting go of limiting beliefs and reaching beyond them to a wider view of yourself and the life you're living.

- "I AM."
- "Through surrendering to what is, I become whole."
- "I choose the power of life."
- "I release the past and experience the joy of the present moment."
- "My thoughts, words, and actions support me."
- "I am worthy to love and be loved."

Releasing the Past

Sometimes as we practice our yoga postures, unexpected emotions can surprise and overwhelm us. Don't let this scare you, as it is an indication that your body is ready to release old cellular memory that it has been holding. Physically, our bodies hold the experiences of our past. Whether they were pleasant or painful memories, our cells store them and they can manifest as anything from muscle tightness to even diseases of the body. Through the combination of your breath, physical movements, and mental focus, these memories begin to dislodge from the subconscious as well as from the cellular level of the body. It is a level of the healing process, which should be nurtured and allowed to release. When these emotions begin to come up, breathe through and surrender into them until they dissipate.

This does not mean that you deny how you feel and push the emotions back into your body, but that you experience them, breathe them, and become aware of how they affect you until they subside. You are then left with a deeper understanding of why and how you hold these feeling in your body and how you can release them in a healthy way.

If you find yourself having trouble putting your emotions into perspective, it may be wise to consult a professional therapist to help you unlock and release them. Although yoga generally instills a sense of contentment and peace in our lives, sometimes if we have deep-seated issues that have not been addressed, we may find ourselves in a period of crisis as we process situations from our past. If you continue with your yoga practice while you work through your challenging issues with a therapist, you will find that the process of healing is much faster and more profound. You will find it easier to let go of the past and live fully in the present moment without fear of the future.

Also, allow yourself those feelings of joy, love, peace, and ecstasy that arise when your heart opens during yoga postures. Again, breathe through these emotions and allow them to fill your body. Notice where you hold happy, joyful feelings. Allowing yourself to experience these loving emotions fully allows you to come alive in your present moment!

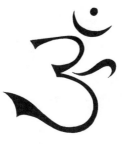

Chapter Seven

The Healing Power of Breath

We can live without food for quite some time. We can even be deprived of water for days before our bodies begin to fail, but we cannot live long at all without breath. Did you know that serious damage can occur when a body has been unable to receive oxygen for only eight minutes?

Breathing is the most important life-supporting action that we do. Without it, nothing else exists. It sustains every system in our body and cleanses impurities from and animates us with life energy, called prana.

Think of a time in your life when you held your breath, waiting for important information. You may have been waiting for an answer regarding your health or the fate of your lost puppy. Now remember how you breathed a sigh of relief when the doctor told you you were fine or when Fluffy came home. Those deep, full breaths helped to relieve the stress you endured during those times of not knowing.

Breathing is the best stress reliever, bar none. It doesn't require any pills or doctor visits. It doesn't need to be stored at room temperature or taken before a certain expiration date. We have a major tool within us that can heal and support our lives. All we have to do is become aware of how we breathe and then inhale and exhale it deeply to begin our healing process. It's simple, it's free, and it's available 100 percent of the time.

Phrases like "a breath of fresh air," or "breathe easy" bring my conscious awareness back to how I inhale and exhale. Sometimes I catch myself holding my breath for no apparent reason. Other times I feel my lungs fill to their greatest capacity as they expand through my whole torso. I have to admit, deep breathing feels much more powerful than the shallow tightness of my chest when I hold my breath. With awareness and practice, let your breath empower and heal you, too.

The Breath of Life

Hatha Yoga, which I introduced in Chapter 6, emphasizes asanas (postures) and pranayama (breath control) to help bring our awareness back to our true Self. In this chapter we will concentrate more fully on our breath and how it can transform our yoga practice as well as our daily life into a state of healing awareness.

It is said that yoga takes the shape of all creation.
—Sri Dharma Mittra, founder of Yoga Asana Center, New York

Our humanness is not what it initially appears to be as a limited, flawed body with the trappings of mental and emotional chatter. As we let go of the material stereotypes of ourselves and breathe into and relax through meditation, yoga postures, and pranayama, we release the boundaries that we draw around ourselves. It is through our breath that we replace these boundaries of our ordinary separate body image with that of our higher Self who is fluid and connected with the larger, all-encompassing whole.

Quantum physics explains that everything is interconnected and that our so-called objective world is an illusion. How, then, can we come to know the truth of who we are if we feel separated within ourselves and among our world? In a word, breath. Our breath and the consciousness we bring to it can shatter our illusions and bring us to the present moment to fully experience the absolute, which is unconditional love.

Pranayama

Pranayama (mindful breathing techniques) helps us focus on physical sensations, allowing our body to become our teacher. Pranayama comes from the root words of "prana," life force, breath, energy, chi; and "ayama," expansion or extension of the life force. As you breathe consciously while you are moving into, holding, or moving out of a posture, you'll enhance the benefits of your practice.

> And the Lord God formed man of the dust of the ground, and breathed into his nostrils the breath of life; and man became a living soul.
> —The Holy Bible, Genesis, 2:7

Correct breathing calms the mind, relaxes the body, strengthens your immune system, and gives you more oxygen. The expansion of the inhalation and the contraction of the exhalation become part of the rhythm of your movement, allowing you to go more deeply into the exercise or meditation.

Deep breathing is one of the major ways we strengthen our nervous system and develop calm and serene minds. Exercises such as meditation, yoga, and tai chi all encourage deep, steady breathing as a way to strengthen the lungs and calm our nerves. Deep breathing of fresh, clean air reaches the core of our stress and helps us to unwind and release the nervous tension we have stored. It also helps to unlock emotional tension.

There are many different types of breath in the practice of pranayama which can be used in different circumstances throughout our life. For example, if you have been exercising and feel a bit overheated, or you are in the middle of an argument with your spouse and can tell you are reaching "the boiling point," you may wish to practice Sitali pranayama (pronounced SEE-ta-lee). This breath helps to cool your emotions as well as your physical body, brain, and nervous system, making it particularly good to do when you are feeling too warm or agitated.

To achieve this breath, roll your tongue into the form of a tube and place your tongue at your lips. Inhale through the tube of your tongue and concentrate on the coolness that you feel at the back of your throat. Hold your breath for a count and then exhale through your nostrils, feeling the coolness spreading throughout your body.

Another helpful pranayama to consider is Nadi Shodhana (alternate nostril breathing), which helps to balance the right and left hemispheres of the brain. If you are feeling unbalanced or unable to focus, this breath can foster mental clarity and deepen your inner awareness by cleansing the stale air from your lungs. It is excellent preparation for meditation.

Practicing this breath requires the alternate closing of your right and left nostrils, corresponding to your inspirations and expirations. Begin by placing your right thumb against your right nostril and breathing through your left nostril. As you complete your inhalation, place your middle fingers from your right hand over your left nostril and exhale through your right nostril. Inhale, again through the right nostril, then close it with your thumb and repeat the sequence as long as you feel comfortable doing so.

I find that when I practice Nadi Shodhana I am able to integrate my left brain thinking with my creative right brain. I don't feel the internal tug-of-war and can relax into the present moment, accepting what is.

I have listed only a small number of pranayama exercises in this book, but there are many more breathing exercises that can help you achieve the benefits of a calm and centered mind, a strong and vibrant body, and balanced emotions. If you are so inclined, I urge you to make a study of pranayama for yourself.

Conscious use of the breath is an invaluable tool for achieving vibrant balance of dynamic focus and relaxed ease. This is where asana practice truly begins.

Physical Effects

Muscles carry memories of every emotion and physical movement of the body. By opening the channels of energy and the chakras that permeate our energetic field, pranayama may bring up deep feelings and physical sensations that at first may seem scary. It is natural for these releases to occur. They need to be physically loosened, stretched out, and then transformed. Deep breathing helps to flush away our old, unconscious thoughts and behavior.

All yoga techniques such as asana, breathing practices, energy locks (bandha), hand positions (mudra), and meditation can be seen as pranayama, because they're all about learning to control our life force. When we practice from this perspective, we'll go much deeper into the techniques. We'll move from doing Hatha Yoga merely from the physical level, into an experience of the essence of what yoga and pranayama are all about: union of our soul with the Divine.

The relationship between our breath and the physical body manifests itself constantly in mundane as well as spiritually uplifting ways. This is to say that we are physically affected as well as spiritually uplifted through the way we breathe.

Think of a time when you received some good news. Perhaps you received your acceptance letter to graduate school, found out you got the promotion at work, or your boyfriend asked you to marry him. In each of these cases, did you notice your first reaction was to take a deep breath and then how energy seemed to move up your spine?

Our breath is filled with oxygen and energy, and when it filters through our bodies we feel physical sensations such as tingling, lightness, even perhaps a warm, melting feeling moving through us. Depending on how much awareness we give to our breath and how deeply we inhale and exhale, we can notice far-reaching, positive physical effects.

Breathing from our diaphragm is an excellent way to release mental and physical tension. It calms our mind and induces a state of relaxation in our body, which also increases our energy level by drawing air into the lower portion of our lungs. The lower lobes of our lungs have the most alveoli (tiny air sacs), and therefore have the greatest ability to extract oxygen from the breath we take in.

Believe it or not, deep, full-body breaths can even give an internal massage to our abdominal organs, thereby improving digestion and assimilation. As you can see, breathing connects the physical body with the emotional and mental bodies. It is a good tool for integration, for when we integrate the systems of our body with the workings of our mind and emotions. We can then integrate our lives with others, thus creating our spiritual experience in human form.

Prana (Life Force)

In the *Upanishads*, the ancient yogic texts, it is stated that life is prana, prana is life. So long as prana remains in the body, there is life. Through life force, we obtain immortality. Prana, then, is equated with consciousness. This text can be translated to mean that through our conscious awareness of the life force within us, we acquire true resolve and the desire to transcend the finite world to achieve immortality.

Consciousness (citta) is connected with the life force indwelling in all beings. Like a bird tied to a string, so is the mind.
—*Yoga-Shikha-Upanishad*, ancient yogic text

This life force that we speak of in yoga is more than an esoteric term that we use to call our breath. Prana is more than the breath. In fact, breath is only the external aspect of prana. It is the manifestation of life force that penetrates and sustains all existence. Prana draws our life force into our body (through inhalation) and generally is thought to be located in the upper half of the trunk, especially in our heart and head. Through regulation of our breath and concentration, we can stimulate and direct our energy to support us more fully in the way we practice yoga on our mats and the way we take our practice into our lives.

Prana is the way we raise our attention within our body toward the crown of our head, which creates more subtle experiences of contemplation, understanding, and surrender. It is when prana flows freely through the body that we feel alive, energetic, and clear-headed. It is the animating force within us. Christianity refers to this as the "breath of God." In other words, prana can be likened to the essence of our soul, and our breath is what sustains this essence.

Ask yourself, what does life force mean to you? How is it that you can think and breathe, make decisions, and move your body? What is it exactly that animates you to exist? These questions may not be so easy to answer, but they give you cause to contemplate your life force, which in turn helps to develop your awareness of it.

Practice: Mindful Breathing

Let's take some time now to bring our awareness to our breath and notice how we are holding our body. It's important to be mindful of ourselves as we experience the activities of our lives. Many times we become so engrossed in our challenges and even our joys that we forget about our physical bodies because we are so consumed with mental thoughts and emotional fluctuations. It can be difficult for us to get into the feelings of our body, and thus we intellectualize most of our experiences. Wouldn't it be wonderful if we could actually "feel" our experiences without having to rationalize them all of the time?

The One breathed, without breath, by Its own power Nothing else was there …
—Hymn of Creation, *The Rig Veda*, oldest and most sacred Hindu scripture

Take some deep inhalations and exhalations and be conscious of where your breath is going. How full are your lungs? How long is your inhale? How long is your exhale? Are you holding your breath at the end of each cycle?

Now, try to remember if you had any thoughts of the past or of the future during the time you were staying conscious of your breath. This awareness will allow you to get back into your physical body, thus connecting it with your mind and emotions instead of alienating it.

You will get the most out of your physical yoga practice by doing this simple exercise. Your breath will help you move deeper into each asana, feeling a greater sense of space, peace, and release. Once you can surrender to your breath on the mat in yoga class, you will find that you will be able to breathe easier in the situations of your life and meet them with grace and poise.

Riding the Waves

Sometimes our lives feel as if we are being rocked back and forth in the middle of an ocean squall. The waves bash against the sides of our little rowboat and we feel like we're drowning in the midst of all our problems, to-do lists, and responsibilities of our life. When things seem so overwhelming that we find it hard to separate ourselves from our problems, we must remember to step back, take a breath, and re-evaluate the situations we find ourselves in. Inevitably, nothing is as bad as it seems at first glance, and by coming back to our centered present, we see clearly how to adjust our attitudes. Without this self-awareness, we would continue in a downward spiral of stress and frustration, separating from our true nature, which is that of unconditional love and pure awareness.

When we can learn to go with the flow of our lives, letting go of trying to control the outcomes of any situation, we will start to feel freer and more able to handle the stress of our lives. So, how do we get from the place of complete chaos to that centered, peaceful place that we hear so much about in yoga?

If we can relax and calm the body, our minds will follow the lead and begin to surrender to a more focused state of being. In turn, when the mind is still, our emotions come into balance. The best way to achieve this fully balanced and centered state within our body/mind/spirit connection is to start with our breath.

Begin by noticing how your breath flows into your body. Feel the waving sensation as you inhale, expanding deeply into the lowest part of your lungs. Feel your breath wash over and heal you. As you exhale, feel that wave move upward and out of your body connecting to the next wave of your breath. Notice how there is no beginning nor ending to your breath, only the ebb and flow are present as you focus on the nurturing, waving motion of prana.

When we can bring our awareness back to the present moment using our breath, we can release the regrets we have from our past. Whether it was missed deadlines, unsaid truths to a loved one, or lost opportunities, we can let go of the guilt that the past holds. Likewise, as we breathe fully into the "now," we can surrender our fear of the unknown future and let go of stress that may be unfounded. We can then ride the waves of our breath to a calm, centered, and relaxed state of being.

I like to think of "riding the waves" as floating weightlessly on clear, turquoise blue water, feeling my breath coincide with the movement of the ocean surf. When trouble starts to overwhelm me, I close my eyes and begin to practice Ujjayi Breath and I visualize myself in the scene of the calm ocean surf. In no time, within just a few rounds of breath, I am able to handle my stress and I can see better possibilities for the future.

Your Breath Is the "Now"

One of the teachings of yoga states that the body signifies the past, the mind signifies the future, and the breath is the present. Therefore, our breath links our body and mind, our past and our future, and brings us into the stillness of the present moment.

Full body breathing is an extraordinary symphony of both powerful and subtle movements that massage our internal organs, oscillate our joints, and alternately tone and release all the muscles in the body. It is a full participation in life.

—Donna Farhi, international yoga instructor and author

Many philosophers and yoga masters say there is no reality except for the "now." We may have memories, but we cannot live in the past. Those experiences are over. We can plan for and fear the idea of our future, but how can we live there if we experience our lives one moment at a time? We can say that we plan for our future by saving money for our children's education, scheduling time off for vacations, making time for our retirement, but we are not living there, we are living a series of present moments hoping that our plans will go according to our wishes. This thinking tends to waste our present and pull us away from the "now" where we truly experience life.

I've recognized when I have slipped out of my present moment awareness and into some thoughts of my past experiences or future hopes when I have stopped breathing regularly. Tension builds in my muscles and in my thoughts until finally I take a deep breath, which pulls me back to my body and into the awareness of the "now." Every time this happens I am amazed that my mind had taken me so far away from the consciousness of my body and the present moment.

Can you think of an instance when you caught yourself holding your breath? What prompted you to inhale? How did you feel after your breaths became regular again?

Pranayama and yoga postures were developed by the ancient sages to release the whirling thoughts of the mind and bring us to stillness so that we may know the unconditional sense of oneness. This understanding is so important in order for us to experience the "now." It is in these moments of present awareness that we experience growth and find our true nature and the essence of unconditional love.

Without present moment awareness, we can become overwhelmed by the many choices we have created and the number of relationships we are in. By using our breath to keep us centered, we focus our mind and stabilize our emotions to see the full picture of our life. At this point we can make conscious decisions and experience our life the way we choose.

Ujjayi Breath

The diaphragm is a large muscle that separates your chest cavity from your abdominal region and is a very important component in helping you breathe. In its relaxed state, it is dome-shaped, which gives the abdominal organs plenty of room. When the diaphragm is contracted, it flattens out, moving downward, pushing the abdomen out at the same time, pulling the lower part of the lungs downward. This movement creates more space for the lungs to expand. It also lowers the air pressure in the lungs, which causes air to rush in to fill the partial vacuum. As you exhale, the diaphragm relaxes and draws upward, back into the dome-shape.

Finally with courage in your heart and God by your side you take a stand, you take a deep breath, and you begin to design the life you want to live as best you can.

—Anonymous

Breathing with your diaphragm is the most effective way of expanding your chest cavity. Most people only use about the first one fourth to one third of their lung capacity and find that they run out of breath easily or they fatigue quickly.

Ujjayi Breath enables us to use our entire lung capacity, therefore filling our body with oxygen and prana (life force energy) at a greater rate. It is often used in conjunction with many different styles of yoga to help practitioners control the flow of breath and therefore calm the mind and heart so as to experience a more focused practice.

You will immediately sense a boost of energy and alertness as well as a sense of calm with your first full Ujjayi Breath. As you continue this breath it will eventually become second nature to you and you will notice greater stamina, more mental clarity, and emotional balance.

Breathing deeply, as with Ujjayi Breath, you may also notice weight loss. This is accomplished through better metabolism due to your increased lung capacity. When you breathe more deeply, you are oxygenating your blood at a much faster rate, which in turn increases the supply of nutrients to your cells and helps to burn excess fat. Ujjayi Breath also has been known to lower high blood pressure in practitioners. The relaxation response from oxygenating our bodies fully relieves the pressure in the circulatory system, thus lowering blood pressure.

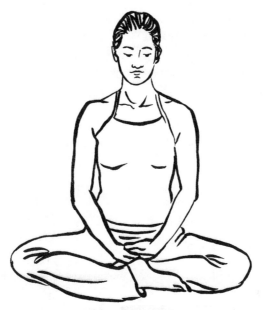

Ujjayi Breath.

Empowerment Exercise: Ujjayi Breath

Ujjayi Breath Affirmation: *I inhale empowerment. I exhale joy!*

The benefits of Ujjayi Breath are profound and time-tested. Allow yourself to take a few moments to breathe Ujjayi pranayama and immediately feel the effects of this healing elixir:

1. Notice your natural breathing pattern (inhale-expand/exhale-soften) and feel how your breath is moving through your throat.

2. Inhale slowly through both nostrils, swallow, and keep your throat slightly constricted near the back of your throat to help you feel and hear your breath. (The sound may remind you of ocean waves and will be audible in your ears.)

3. Your exhale should flow through the nostrils.

4. Notice how the breath fills your lungs, feeling the belly expand first, then feel the chest expanding easily until you have reached the end of your inhale.

5. On your exhale, let the belly soften and drop first, then allow the chest to soften. Your breaths should be deep, long, and full.

6. End Ujjayi Breath after a long exhalation and allow your breath to find its normal pace once again. Become aware of your normal breath and notice how it has changed.

Benefits

The most important benefit of Ujjayi Breath is life force. We can't live without it! Through our breath, fresh oxygen and energy enter our bodies and clear out the stale air from our lungs. Our breath oxygenates our blood, heart, and brain, and in turn improves our immune system and increases our lung capacity.

The benefits continue throughout our bodies by increasing energy, releasing mental and physical tension, improving our moods, soothing our nervous system, and giving us a profound sense of peace and well-being. Ujjayi Breath also internally massages our abdominal organs, improves digestion, and releases blocked energy that can cause physical disease.

Ujjayi Breath also affects the third and fourth chakras by expanding through our torsos and chests. The corresponding chakras relate to self-esteem, confidence, and personal power (third chakra) as well as love, compassion, kindness, and peace (fourth chakra). This pranayama has also been known to help relieve asthma, allergies, high blood pressure, and coronary troubles.

If you do no other type of yoga except practice Ujjayi Breath every day, you will feel the most profound changes throughout your body, mind, and emotions. Throughout my teaching career, I have had students proudly announce to me that through practicing Ujjayi Breath, they have lowered their blood pressure, made 100 percent scores on tests, relieved migraine headaches, and even focused their wandering minds.

Without breath our physical bodies cannot exist. Ujjayi Breath allows us to inspire the most amount of energy from the oxygen we breathe, which in turn purifies our entire system, expelling diseases and negative energy.

Cautions

There are no real dangers in practicing Ujjayi Breath; however, if you breathe too fast, you may begin to feel lightheaded. Hyperventilation is rare but can happen if you are not mindful with the practice.

Be cautious if practicing this breath while driving an automobile. If you feel lightheaded, stop Ujjayi Breath and relax your throat to breathe in a normal, deep inhalation, then exhale it slowly and let your breath move back to its normal rhythm.

As you become more adept with the practice of Ujjayi Breath, you will find that lightheadedness will become infrequent but the benefits of a clear mind and relaxed body will increase.

Real Life

Some of my students visit with me after classes and share their experiences with me regarding how their yoga practice has affected their lives. A woman who looked vaguely familiar to me came up after an evening class and asked if I remembered her. She explained her profound life change with this account of breath:

"My husband and I started taking yoga together just about six months ago. It was a new experience for us and we both felt immediate benefits from the first class we took. We had planned to continue with our newfound practice until my husband suddenly fell ill and had to have emergency surgery twice. With numerous trips to the hospital and long stays each time, neither one of us could make it back to another yoga class.

I spent all my time at his side, trying to comfort and do all I could to ease his pain. I felt so helpless. During that time, one thing kept coming back to me even though I completely abandoned any kind of exercise routine. 'Breathe, breathe.'

As I spent more and more time in the hospital with my husband I realized I would forget to breathe! Then I would remember the words of our yoga teacher, '… deep, full breaths … feel the breath flow into your lungs …' Immediately I would take a deep breath and become more aware of how I breathed. I was even able to remind my husband to breathe during those times when his pain was so severe, which helped him to relax.

I truly believe I was able to handle my husband's illness in part because of that one class and my new experience with breathing. I also believe that it helped my husband navigate through the difficulty of his illness. I am forever changed by one little word and one huge experience … 'breathe.'"

Empowerment Journal

As you can see from reading the following portion of Yvonne's empowerment journal, yoga not only makes our body fit and stronger, but it helps to ward off germs and disease by strengthening our immune system.

It's also impressive and important to note that yoga is not just for the young but also the young at heart. People of all ages come to this practice and everyone has reaped some benefit. It is never too late to start living and loving what you do in life!

For 63 years I had enjoyed good health when all of a sudden I began having yearly bouts with pneumonia. My lifestyle of healthy diet and regular exercise had begun to fall short in helping me withstand the yearly illness.

At 67, with the purpose of maintaining and enhancing my flexibility, I enrolled in a weekly yoga class. I am now 68 and have been practicing for about a year with no recurring symptoms of pneumonia. I am even feeling physically stronger and younger! What started out as a physical ed. class to help keep my body flexible and fit turned into a life-changing experience of radiant health and a greater quality of life. I have more energy and creativity. Because my body feels better, I feel better and really am grateful for my discovery of yoga breathing and postures.

Mantras for Daily Living

Using a mantra to remind us to take deep, full breaths is helpful, especially for those times when we get so caught up in the experiences of our daily routines that we forget ourselves. Isn't it odd that we are so busy doing things in our life for other people, taking care of our family, making sure our boss is pleased with our work, doing favors for our friends, that there doesn't seem to be any room left in our own life for ourselves? These are the times we most need a reminder to breathe and make space for ourselves.

When you feel your muscles tightening in your shoulders and you become mentally agitated, remind yourself to breathe by reciting your personal mantra. As you inhale, say your mantra, and on your exhalation, say your mantra. Instill the power of your words as you breathe deeply with the pranayamas you've learned in this chapter.

Take a look at the following suggestions and see if any of them resonate with you. You may find one of your own that has a deeper meaning for you. Either way, the recitation of your mantra will remind your cellular memory to relax, breathe, and let go! When you can remember to breathe on such a deep level in your body, then it becomes automatic and you can fully experience prana, your life force.

- "Breathe! Just breathe."
- "The breath of life flows through me like a wave."
- "I breathe in lightness and health."
- "Breathe in, breathe out."
- "My breath animates my Spirit."
- "I am peaceful. I am calm."

"Just Breathe!"

In me I have found only one reality; that I breathe in and I breathe out. And so anything that breathes in or out is a reality. When I found this as a reality in everybody, I found myself in everybody and everybody in myself.

—Yogi Bhajan, Master of Kundalini Yoga, founder of 3HO (Happy, Healthy, Holy Organization)

There is a scene in the movie *Ever After* where Drew Barrymore is preparing to enter the ball and meet her Prince Charming face to face and tell him who she really is. As their eyes meet from across the room, she whispers to herself, "breathe, just breathe." Like Drew's character in the movie, we must remind ourselves to breathe, to keep the flow of our energy moving through us so we can fully participate in the reality of our lives.

Can you remember a time when you had to remind yourself to breathe? I was a sophomore in high school and ready to enter stage right to act in my very first drama. Standing in the wings I could feel my legs shaking as I went over and over the two lines I had in the play. The thought of standing in front of an audience of hundreds of people and forgetting my lines just terrified me.

I was getting more and more anxious as my cue came closer when one of my fellow actors, a senior veteran, came up next to me, put her arm around me and said, "Breathe, you're gonna be great." She snapped me out of it! I realized at that moment what I was doing to myself. Holding my breath, depriving my body of oxygen, and tensing my muscles was definitely not conducive to relaxation. I started to breathe again, just in time to walk onstage, say my lines, and stand on my mark until the curtain closed.

We come to the realization that our breath is most important to our physical existence and through the various pranayama techniques we have been given by the ancient yogis, we can heal ourselves in body, mind, and spirit. Our breath integrates the body and mind as well as connects our past and future with the present moment.

While breathing is an important physical component in our existence, prana is more than that. It is more than oxygen, more than inhalation and exhalation, more than our breath. It is our life force, the animating property that allows us to think and feel and experience life from a higher consciousness. Through our breath, we receive this life force upon every inspiration and expiration, which allows us to handle the ups and downs of our lives from a calm, centered place.

All we have to remember to experience the healing powers of pranayama is to "just breathe!"

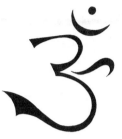

Chapter Eight

Celebration of Your Spirit

When we came to this earth as infants, we were pure, authentic, and whole. Our spirits were free and boundless. We were open to all possibilities through unconditional love and pure consciousness, which is our spiritual essence and our true nature.

Somehow, though, as we grew into adulthood our true nature got covered up with mounds of guilt and blankets of self-consciousness. We forgot to keep an inward focus and trust that our intuition would always guide us. Instead, we found ourselves looking outward to others for answers, trusting someone else's opinion more than we trusted our own.

I'm not saying that we can't trust others, but what is important is that we trust our inner Self, beyond anything external. Spending time turning inward is the greatest act of consciousness and the most self-loving thing we can do for ourselves. So, here we start to celebrate our Spirit, to focus our awareness inward, and to honor the great, beautiful, loving, kind, brilliant beings that we are.

Pratyahara

Pratyahara, meaning withdrawal of the senses, is one of the components that help to complete the Yoga Sutras, and thus bring the yoga practitioner to enlightenment. At first glance it does not seem like an easy path to follow when you consider withdrawing your senses from outside stimuli.

Let's face it, we all love to experience the world around us by watching a good movie, eating popcorn at that movie, sharing conversations with friends, and even enjoy working out at the gym, or taking our weekly yoga classes. Does this mean that we have to give all of that up in order to follow the path of pratyahara? Although the ancient yogic texts seem very strict and unyielding in some aspects, it was not ultimately meant that we forsake our physical and energetic bodies just for the mind. After all, yoga is about integration and honoring all aspects of the Self.

In pratyahara, we shift our awareness from the exploration and cleansing of our external world, our physical body, to the exploration and cleansing of our internal world, the mind, and our intuitive sense. For our modern world, this means that we make time for ourselves, looking deep within, understanding our motivations, our fears, our hopes and desires, everything. This is the place were we see ourselves in full light, good and bad, strong and weak, with the understanding that everything that we are is ultimately for our benefit. It is through the negative aspects of ourselves that we are challenged to grow into enlightenment.

Through this cultivation of inward concentration we can then release outside distractions of sight and sound and develop our inner senses of these experiences. The wisdom of the *Shvetashvatara-Upanishad* (3:19) states, "sees without eyes, hears without ears." This is what we seek to achieve when we practice withdrawing our senses from the outside world, to see past the physical sight and hear more clearly than physical sounds. We strengthen our sixth chakra of intuition so we see and hear from a more expanded awareness.

The phrase "can't see the forest for the trees" has much more wisdom than we think. If we can't see the forest because of all the trees, that must mean then that we are too distracted with all the things around us in our lives. It is difficult to step outside of the bombardment of sights and sounds so we can witness the whole experience, but this is precisely what we have to do to trust our intuition and remember our true Self.

How, then, can we withdraw our senses from all the distractions of our life? You're probably thinking that because you may have a spouse and children to tend to, and a job that requires much of your time, that this discipline of pratyahara is not for you. Before you dismiss this important tool for your enlightenment, take a little closer look at how we of the modern age can adapt pratyahara to our busy lives and, in turn, reawaken our true nature.

Turning Inward

Turning inward is another name for personal reflection. I'm wondering if you just held your breath at the thought of maybe having to do some soul searching! I admit that looking inside ourselves can be a little frightening. No one really wants to look at the shadow side of themselves. As we've grown up, it's been mentioned to us on many occasions that "we must be good," or "don't cry in public," or the best line, "no one will like you if you do this or that ...." Well, that's enough to scare anyone away from truly taking a good look inside and finding out what's really there.

> The student has hindsight; the teacher has foresight; the master has insight ... you are here to become a student, a teacher and a master-one who learns from the past, foresees the consequences of your actions, and finally, looks within to discover the Universe.
>
> —Dan Millman, author of *Way of the Peaceful Warrior*

The key to finding the courage to look inward is to stop worrying about what other people think of you. Stop believing in others' assumed notions of who you are and trust your own perceptions about your innate worthiness. This is what pratyahara is all about. Withdraw your senses from the casual, uninformed perceptions of other people and turn inward to your own truth. Stop seeing *your* world through someone else's eyes and discover life's gifts and opportunities. You will receive this abundance according to how you see your own self-worth.

Our society's conditioning can be threatening to our body/mind/spirit health, but it doesn't have to mean that we stay stuck in our ruts and ignore what's happening on the inside of our real Self. Let your yoga practice release you from outside influences. While you are on your mat, be there and nowhere else. Breathe into your body and move through the postures as if you are each posture.

It is much easier to approach our daily routines when we have taken the time to turn inward through the movements of our bodies in yoga.

Detachment

Many of us have the idea that detachment is only related to disinterest or even depression. Yoga takes this term more deeply into the spiritual realm where we are able to see how important and healthy it is for us to be detached from the outcome of a situation. The attachment to things, situations, and even people pulls us away from our calm internal center and dilutes our focus and energy outward.

In detachment lies the wisdom of uncertainty … in the wisdom of uncertainty lies the freedom from the known, which is the prison of past conditioning.
—Deepak Chopra, best-selling author and physician

In order to manifest or achieve anything in our lives, we have to let go of our attachment to it. This doesn't mean that we have to give up our intentions for what we want nor do we have to lose our desire for our goal, but we must give up our attachment to the result. In other words, we must be detached from the ways our intentions and desires are met. When we can relinquish our attachment to the result, we become free from fear and control and we begin to feel more creative and joyful.

Attachment is based on fear and insecurity and the need for security is based on not knowing our true Self. Once we know who we are internally, we are freer to accept our reality as it is. Detachment, then, is a key component in letting go of the need to have things be as we think they should be. Without detachment we become overwhelmed with the feelings of helplessness, hopelessness, and trivial concerns which pull us so far away from our calm center that it is difficult to surrender.

At times I've come to a yoga class in a rush, either pushed by traffic or by my own procrastination and tardiness, which made me start my practice feeling a little on edge. My mind got left somewhere between the highway and class, which meant that my postures reflected my unbalanced internal self—until, that is, I let go in my mind of the events that occurred before I got to class. Once I became fully present on my mat, nothing else mattered. I detached from the past and surrendered to the uncertainty of the future. Each posture that I attempted then became a graceful movement that flowed through my body and my breath.

Can you think of a time when you released your attachment to something and how it felt as you let go? One of my students, Alison, shared with me a perfect example of using yoga in helping her to detach from a situation and create a peaceful center. She explained, "I remember one night, early in my yoga practice, I was lying in bed and feeling a rush of anxiety, afraid that I couldn't fall asleep. Then I heard my own breathing and somehow my breath helped me to let go of my fear of not falling asleep and I began to feel centered, peaceful, and supported. I fell asleep in no time."

In uncertainty we find the freedom to create anything because we are not attached to an idea, an outcome or even the security we think it provides. In reality, the search for security is an illusion and also an attachment to the known, which keeps us on that merry-go-round of fear and anxiety. When we experience uncertainty, and can detach from it, we can know that we are on the right path.

The next time you find yourself getting upset about a situation that you don't seem to have control over, detach yourself from the outcome and see what happens to your mood. Tell yourself it doesn't matter what happens in the situation and that either way, you'll be fine and things will work out. If you have to, try some deep breathing or fold into a forward bend for a few seconds to help your body connect with what your mind is telling yourself.

When you force solutions you only create more problems. Witness the uncertainty while you expectantly wait for the solution to emerge out of the chaos. Through this detachment you will find yourself letting go of outside problems and turning inward to your calm centered oasis.

Taking Time for Yourself

It has never been easier to get in touch with people all over the planet with just the push of a few buttons. The Internet and cell phones can put us in contact with loved ones or a business associate within seconds, even if they live across town, across the country or across the world. Technology is truly amazing, but is it allowing us as human beings to truly experience ourselves? It seems that everywhere I look lately someone is on his/her cell phone. It doesn't matter if they're having dinner with friends, driving in their car, or even taking a hike in the middle of the woods! As much as I marvel at our ability to communicate with others because of our electronic devices, I am concerned about how we communicate with ourselves these days. Where is the downtime for us to sit for a few moments and contemplate life? How long as it been since we actually evaluated our happiness?

> Like two golden birds perched on the selfsame tree, intimate friends, the ego and the Self dwell in the same body. The former eats the sweet and sour fruits of the tree of life, while the latter looks on in detachment.
> —*Mundaka Upanishad*, ancient yogic text

Our communication devices have turned into a sort of double-edged sword in that they are a great help when it comes to staying in touch, but they have now blurred the boundaries of work and relaxation, of external awareness versus internal understanding.

In American society we think of our lives as "work." We spend most of our free time finding ways to cut corners, accomplishing more and increasing production while we forget about playing, relaxing, and getting to know ourselves and others in a more intimate way. In a sense, I wonder if we are dehumanizing ourselves.

For example, a CEO of a prestigious company is getting ready to surprise his wife with a weekend trip to the seashore for their first anniversary. He solidifies all the plans on his cell phone on his drive home from the office. He's thought of everything and has even packed their bags ahead of time so he can just come home and whisk her away! It sounds romantic, doesn't it?

It's 3 P.M. on a Friday, he gets home, surprises his honey, and within the hour they are on their way to the ocean for a wonderful vacation together. All is running smoothly until his cell phone rings—it's the office telling him there's a problem at work and he's the only one who can fix it. (Keep in mind, it's a Friday and by this time it's well after the workday should be complete.) Our prince charming has two choices: One, he turns the car around and heads back to the city to take care of a problem that probably could have been fixed without him and loses the time with his wife. Two, he tells the office he's out of town and can't come back, but he feels guilty during the rest of his weekend and his first anniversary gets blurred in his memory.

Perhaps the better choice would have been to leave the cell phone at home or at least turned off during their trip. This gesture is saying that he acknowledges himself and his wife and their need for intimacy and rest. They are taking time for themselves. At that moment, they are more important to each other than any business or problem. The boundaries have been clearly set and everyone knows where they stand.

This example may look like I'm against cell phones, but I don't mean it to sound that way. I actually like cell phones and have one myself, but I believe there are responsible ways of using them so we can live each of our present moments to the fullest.

There have been times in the yoga classes that I teach that someone's cell phone will go off right in the middle of class, or worse yet, in Savasana when everyone is letting go into relaxation! It's during those moments that the whole class takes a deep breath, the owner of the cell phone turns it off and whispers an apology and I make a mental note to announce in the next class, "turn off all cell phones!"

Taking time for ourselves has become a lost art and with it our sense of who we really are has been hidden from our view. Even if we take a few moments each day to breathe mindfully or practice a couple of yoga postures, we are re-establishing the link back to ourselves. It is in knowing ourselves that we make conscious and intelligent decisions within our lives.

Practice: Alone Time

Have you ever noticed your friends apologizing for not keeping in touch better because they are "too busy" with their lives? I am even guilty of telling this to my friends and family. It makes me stop and ask the question, "What am I really busy with?" As I turn inward and restate the question, I find that most of my busyness can be eliminated or at least be re-arranged so that I can fit into my own life better.

Resolve to be thyself: and know, that he who finds himself, loses his misery.
—Matthew Arnold, English critic, essayist, and poet

When I do my morning yoga practice and meditation, I find that I have enough time in a day to accomplish more than what I set out to do. It is the times that I skimped on or missed my practice altogether that I felt rushed and out of time. Yoga and meditation are the best stress reliefs I know of to help turn my thoughts inward and let go of outside distractions.

For our practice, we are going to spend some "alone time." If we ever hope to slow down, enjoy meaningful connections, live life consciously and feel true love, we must find the time to spend alone.

Start with 10 minutes out of your day and shut the door to your office, turn off the phones, or step outside and sit under a tree. It doesn't matter where you go as long as you are alone. Take some deep, full breaths, filling your lungs as deeply as you can, and then exhale slowly, noticing how your body feels as you release the air. Turn your thoughts inward and ask yourself the question, "Am I happy here and now?" and wait for your answer.

Eventually, extend your alone time to an hour, half of a day, even a whole weekend depending on your schedule, and really get to know yourself, understanding what motivates you. As your alone time becomes longer, use it to do a silent yoga practice. Feel the physical sensations of your body and listen to your mind and emotions. Breathe a sigh of surrender as you come to know yourself more intimately.

Intuition

Intuition is the essence of the sixth chakra. It is that still small voice inside us, and sometimes honoring women as a "woman's intuition." We've been told to trust it and we've also been told that it isn't reliable because there is no solid evidence that it exists. I'm sure many people who actually do trust that small voice inside can give plenty of examples to show that, in fact, intuition is a viable and necessary part of who we are.

> Your subconscious holds keys to a treasure house of intuitive wisdom, clear sight, and untapped power. All you have to do is to look, listen, and trust, paying attention to dreams, feelings and instinct.
> —Dan Millman, author of *Way of the Peaceful Warrior*

Also known as our sixth sense, intuition is that voice in our head that says, from out of the blue, "turn around and look down." You do just in time to sidestep a hole in the sidewalk avoiding a fall. It also is that hunch that makes you stop at a store out of the way on your route home from work only to run into a friend you've been thinking about and haven't seen in years!

Can you remember the time when you first met your spouse and you said to yourself "I'm going to marry her" because you just knew it? Later, you thought "This is crazy, how can I know this about love so soon?" As it turned out, you've been married for years and still feel like she's the one. My sister did exactly that. She dated her husband for a few months but she said she knew he was the one for her from their second date. They've been married for 15 years now and still act like two peas in a pod.

Intuition is much more than odd little magical instances that amaze us every time they occur. It is perception beyond our physical senses and the voice of our higher Self. It is the understanding of the whole of our consciousness beyond our physical awareness.

Have you ever had someone on your mind so strongly that you couldn't stop thinking about them, only to run into them unexpectedly or receive a call from them? Maybe you knew the phone was going to ring a split second before it did and you knew who was calling before you even picked up the phone and checked caller ID. These are all examples of our intuition and how we actually are connected to all beings.

During my yoga classes, we practice being open to our intuition on the mat. Through our breath and movement and through the postures, we learn to trust the thoughts and feelings that come to us. Intuition is a very subtle yet profound experience, and it is important to be open to whatever we are feeling or sensing, or whatever thoughts come to us. However, it is also important to distinguish between the thoughts we create ourselves and the intuitive voice that speaks to us from a greater consciousness.

You may wonder how you can tell the difference between your regular thoughts and your intuition. The simple truth is that we must listen with more than our ears. We must listen with our whole physical body, mental body, and emotional body. Yoga is one of the best ways I know for increasing our intuition and decreasing all the extraneous mind chatter that we sometimes confuse for our intuition. When we hold a pose, breathing through it, concentrating only on our breath and feeling the effects in our body, mind and emotions, we are opening ourselves up to hear our intuition.

Perhaps you are drawn to Virabhadrasana (Warrior Pose, see Chapter 5) for example, and you practice it daily for a few weeks, more so than the poses of your regular routine. You're not sure why, but it "feels good" to practice this particular pose at this time.

The Warrior Pose is a pose of strength and courage. It relates to an inner strength and resolve as well as strengthening our foundation and centering our core. Ask yourself if you've felt the need to fortify your life in this manner. Perhaps you've needed a little more courage to approach your boss for that well-deserved and overdue raise, or maybe you're contemplating "popping the question" to your girlfriend but you're feeling a fear of commitment or rejection starting to creep into your thoughts. You might even be needing a little more resolve to follow through on the commitment you made to yourself to quit smoking. In either case, the Warrior Pose has fortified you with courage to withstand the illusion of doubt and fear that your thoughts can sometimes create. Intuitively, you knew that this pose would help and your body naturally moved in this direction.

The next time you practice yoga, pay attention to the poses you gravitate toward and the ones that really empower you. Notice the feelings the pose creates within you and ask yourself how you can apply them to your daily life. Through yoga your body is expressing the intuition of your higher Self. We must listen to our bodies, it is an excellent tool to help us become more aware of that still, small voice within that guides us to greater knowledge and higher awareness. It leads us to compassion for ourselves and others as well, it brings us to a calm, trusting state which makes us even more accepting of the intuitive thoughts and feelings that speak to us on a regular basis.

Aloneness vs. Loneliness

Being alone and loneliness don't necessarily have to accompany each other. Many people have a difficult time being alone and thus feelings of loneliness ensue because they don't know how to entertain themselves. But ultimately, being alone is much more empowering than the feeling of loneliness that can sometimes accompany our solitary time.

The definition of alone relates to either being by oneself or being exclusive or unequaled. That definition doesn't give any indication of sadness or feeling unempowered. As a matter of fact, considering ourselves to be unequaled can be quite empowering. We are unequalled in the talents and abilities that we alone have. Ultimately, there is no one else in this world like you, like me, like the guy down the street. We are all exclusively unique in who we are and what we have to offer to the world, yet we all share the same connection of Spirit.

When we share ourselves and our gifts for the advancement of our higher Self and that of the human experience, then we are fulfilled and even in our aloneness we are enriched; however, we are never lonely because we are giving of ourselves.

Loneliness, on the other hand, is the feeling of isolation and depression from feeling the lack of companionship. It is the fear of feeling you are alone, separate or cut off from your source of happiness, protection, or your security. Feeling lonely is related to our first chakra, our center of foundation and security. If you find that you are feeling a little cut off from your family and friends, even yourself, you may be experiencing a weakened root chakra. When you are feeling lonely, ask yourself if you are feeling grounded. Do you feel secure with your career, your relationships, your life? If you realize these issues are part of your depression or loneliness, try doing yoga postures that support your foundation. The most reliable and easiest to do is Tadasana (Mountain Pose, see Chapter 1). Stand up straight, ground into your feet and legs, relax your buttocks. This helps you to let go of physical and mental stress of holding on to fear.

Another area that affects our feelings of loneliness is our fourth energy center, the heart chakra. Our chest, lungs, and heart are where we hold feelings of love, compassion, and acceptance. When our heart center is negatively affected, feelings of grief and sadness get stuck in our heart chakra as well. These emotions can cause depression and loneliness.

To clear the loneliness, heart postures are important. Try backward-bending poses, which help to open and stimulate your heart. Bring yourself to Ustrasana (Camel Pose, see Chapter 4) and notice how the emotions begin to release. After a series of heart-opening postures, you most likely will notice you are feeling lighter in your heart and the loneliness is either gone or greatly reduced.

Spending time alone is important to our internal awareness and our self-empowerment. It is a time for contemplation and re-evaluation. It is a time to look squarely into the mirror of ourselves and accept our reality. Through being alone, we can put things into perspective. We can make conscious decisions regarding our health, our work, and our relationships. Sometimes in our aloneness we don't have to do anything, we don't have to plan anything, and we don't even have to think about anything. Being alone affords us the awareness of just "being."

I have found as I have grown older that my alone time has become increasingly valuable. I enjoy spending time alone with myself more now than I ever did when I was younger. This time by myself rejuvenates me, helps me to organize my thoughts and schedules, but mostly it allows me to get to know myself better and feel more comfortable in my own skin. Thanks to my time alone, I am able to be much more present with my family, friends, and my students in class. Through taking the time to be alone, I have realized what I like in my life and what I wish to release from my life. I have actually realized that I like myself. It's a beautiful thing when you like yourself, because when you do, loneliness doesn't knock on your door very often. If you truly like your own company, you always have a friend, a confidant, and a companion along your journey.

Ultimately, the big difference between being alone and loneliness is fear, which emotionally isolates us from our friends, family, and mostly from our Divine nature, God. When we connect to our higher Self, listen to our inner voice (which can clearly be heard when we are alone), we are never lonely but find moments of great peace and insight in our aloneness.

Parvatasana (Seated Mountain Pose)

Parvatasana is a powerful affirmation of inner strength. This graceful and surprisingly intense posture can bring us to a grounded center unlike any we've known. Not only does it ground us fully into our present moment, it helps to raise our energy up through our heart and crown. The prayer hangs over our head, directs this energy, and lifts it upward in a focused way, which directs our intention upward and our attention inward. In this position, our hands also act like an energy conductor focusing prana back to us.

In a sense, in Parvatasana we are becoming a channel for energy to move through us and into us from the Universal Mind, or God. Parvatasana expresses prayer in the physical form. Through its dynamic gesture toward the heavens, it incorporates the body and mind in our prayer.

It affects all seven energy centers from our root chakra through our crown chakra. By first grounding into our seated position, we are stimulating our first and second chakras. As we raise our hands above our head and breathe deeply, expanding into the solar plexus, stretching through the chest, and focusing toward our third eye, we have stimulated our power center, our heart, and our intuitive center. Finally, with our hands over head in prayer, we are directing our focus and energy through the crown of our head, thus stimulating our seventh chakra and opening to the awareness of God within us, of our higher Self, and of greater consciousness. By incorporating deep, full breaths with this posture, it becomes intensely energetic and transformative.

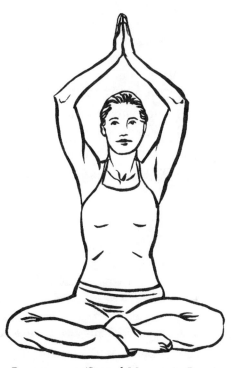

Parvatasana (Seated Mountain Pose).

Empowerment Exercise: Parvatasana

Parvatasana Affirmation: *I reach to heaven with an open heart.*

Parvatasana can be practiced every day to increase mental focus and increase upper body strength. It is an unobtrusive yet powerful asana.

1. Begin by sitting in Siddhasana (Perfect Pose, see Chapter 10) with your hands, palms facing upward, on your knees.

2. Inhale and circle your hands overhead, bring your palms together in a prayer, and lengthen through your spine to create space between your vertebrae.

3. Exhale and soften your elbows slightly, relaxing your shoulders down your back.

4. Inhale and draw your abdomen in strongly toward the spine to seal in the breath in your upper torso. Keep your shoulders and chest open, continuing to lift from the crown of your head as you hold your breath. (Begin holding your breath for three counts and progressively hold it for longer periods of time as is comfortable for you.)

5. Repeat for as long as you feel comfortable.

6. To exit, inhale and stretch tall through your spine, then exhale and open your arms out to your sides and lower the hands back to your knees, palms facing upward.

Benefits

Like the Mountain Pose in Chapter 1, Parvatasana focuses on grounded balance; however, it moves our awareness upward and more into our chest and shoulders. This posture increases strength and flexibility in our shoulders, helping to open our breathing space. When our shoulders are more flexible, we then have the ability to move more freely through our torsos, which helps to unlock blocked emotional energy.

Combining the feeling of stability with concentrated awareness in our chest, we experience a dynamic flow of energy upward, toward our third eye, which stimulates our sixth chakra, our intuitive center. This simple little pose heightens the awareness of prana (life force) in our bodies and supports a deep spiritual focus.

Cautions

As you attempt Parvatasana, be aware of your shoulders and knees. If your shoulders are particularly tight, begin by holding a strap in both hands as you lift your arms over your head. This will allow your shoulders to open at their own pace and will not compromise the lift in your spine. Parvatasana should not be done with a rounded spine.

When beginning Parvatasana and entering the cross-legged position, be sure not to twist or rotate your knees. Let the rotation come from the hip joints. If you find that your hips are tight and tend to torque your knees, sit on a cushion or thickly folded blanket to tip your hips forward and thus relieve pressure on your lower back and knees.

You are, when all is said and done—just what you are.
—Goethe, German playwright and novelist

Real Life

I think this sample of real life is priceless! This anonymous student isn't afraid to see and admit what is going on with himself. He truly practices being the witness by observing his weakness and seeing what he has to improve upon. This approach to Self is very wise and compassionate. I commend him for his honest look at reality and for taking responsibility for his choices and experiences.

"Oh, man, the Seated Mountain is not as easy as it looks! The biggest thing I realized about this pose is that my shoulders are tight and I can't sit up straight when my arms are above my head! It looks like I have some work to do.

I have to admit that I'm a little frustrated today because I couldn't do it the way I wanted, but after I finished the pose, and my arms were at my sides, my whole upper body got this rush of … something, tingling, energy … something! That was really cool. I actually felt better *after* I did this pose than while I was doing it. I'm sure I'll get better with practice.

Since I'm pretty new to yoga, I can't really say how it has changed my life, but I guess I have noticed that I have more energy when I'm finished with class and at the same time it's not like a forceful energy, but a quiet, powerful kind of feeling. I really like that part of my practice and wish it would stay with me longer after class. I'm hoping it will last longer the more I take yoga.

In the meantime, I want to keep practicing and see where this takes me."

Empowerment Journal

Wendy is one of my students in Tennessee who truly takes her yoga practice seriously and incorporates it into her life, experiencing true joy and enlightenment. She is dedicated to expanding her consciousness, and at the same time she exists in the "now" without judging her past or fearing her future.

Discovering your worth sets your spirit free!
—Dan Millman, author of *Way of the Peaceful Warrior*

I love this example from her empowerment journal. She has taken a full look at her life and how it has changed since beginning her practice of yoga. You can clearly see the process Wendy has moved through to reach her understanding of what yoga is to her body, mind, and spirit.

This example is the embodiment of yoga. It shows the process we hope to achieve in our practice through introspection, and it proves to us that it indeed is possible to transcend the ego and rise to higher states of consciousness and joy.

Here are some thoughts Wendy shared with me regarding yoga in her life:

I've practiced Hatha Yoga for eight years. It's difficult to say what yoga means to me because I have moved through so many phases in the practice and continue to grow with it as yoga is not so much a goal as it is a journey that lasts a lifetime and then some.

It's like breathing. The practice is in the marrow of my bones now. I'm deeply aware when I experience an emotion or a mood. I know what part of my body is hurting, or if my mind is just full of monkey thoughts. I now have the tools to bring the emotions, moods, physical aches and pains, and mind chatter back into balance whether through my breath, meditation, or postures.

I live my life more in the present now, knowing that the present moment is really the only one we have. I have also experienced more courage and proactive involvement in life as some of the postures and breathing exercises specifically gear themselves to these qualities.

Before discovering yoga I did not enjoy exercising very much. Now, with newfound energy I am enjoying walking, cycling, and hiking through the nature trails where I live. Before yoga I was scarcely aware that I had a body, let alone I didn't like it very much. I now thoroughly delight in the sheer physicality of yoga and witnessing with amazement what my body can do after eight years. I now have a healthy sense of my body, and take care of it nutritionally and otherwise.

Recently, my spouse and I were introduced to partner yoga. We have already felt the benefits of the practice. We are more in sync with each other and more sensitive to each other's needs. It's better than counseling and a lot more fun! What I learn and experience on the mat I take out with me into my life.

Mantras for Daily Living

Have you ever gotten a word or a phrase or the line of a song stuck in your head and it kept repeating over and over again? Sometimes it felt positive and the repetition seemed to empower you and put a spring in your step. Other times, that darn word or phrase sounded like a broken record and no matter what you were doing it seemed to infiltrate your thoughts!

At every single moment of one's life one is what one is going to be no less than what one has been.

—Oscar Wilde, English poet and playwright

I can tell you that this has happened to me many different times when I did not consciously pay attention to my thoughts. Mantras are words, phrases, and even musical phrases that we consciously instill throughout our being to focus our intentions and to help manifest our dreams and desires. The difference between mantras and random thoughts is intention and inward focus.

It's time again to find a mantra that feels right for you regarding coming to your inner awareness. Sometimes single words can be most effective to help bring you inward and release the outside chatter. Words that I find helpful for this practice are *peace, consciousness, witness, breathe,* and *OM,* to name a few.

Think about what turning inward means to you and you may come up with some of your own words and phrases. In the meantime, you are welcome to choose any of these examples to help you with your practice.

- "I AM, that AM."
- "I honor my Divine Spirit."
- "My life is a celebration."
- "I am divinely guided."
- "I trust my intuition."
- "All is well in my world."

Living from the Inside Out

Authenticity is what comes to mind when I think of living my life from the inside out. It means to be genuine and real. We can only see reality clearly when we are clear enough within ourselves to witness the world around us and know that we are in the world but not of the world. In remembering the practice of pratyahara as withdrawing our senses from the external world to strengthen our internal world of intuition and the mind, we can see how important it is for us to know our true Self through spending time alone and introspection. Through these actions we may approach our external world with detachment, and thus experience our life in a more fulfilled, joyful, and productive way.

> It matters not what you are thought to be, but what you are.
> —Publilius Syrus, Latin writer

Our yoga practice is an excellent tool for us to apply to our lives in that it puts our focus in the present moment and integrates our mind and body so we become more conscious in our daily lives. We can experience life from within ourselves, rather than feeling as if we are being thrown about by the challenges we face in our external world.

Earlier in the chapter I introduced you to Alison. I would like to share a little more of her story to help us see how integral our yoga practice in class really is to our everyday life. Her story is personal, but I'm sure every one of us can find threads of this story relating to our own lives:

I was experiencing a lot of anxiety last winter when a friend recommended I try taking a yoga class. Considering how high-strung and prone to panic attacks I am, I gave it a try.

That very first class, the instructor opened by saying "Be in this room, right now, in your body." She told us we didn't have to think about anything else for the next hour. I thought she was talking directly to me. I don't know how it happened, but doing that class calmed me. I felt like that hour was an oasis in the midst of my anxiety, so I kept going back. I knew that no matter how bad my day was, the yoga would be an hour of peace.

Amazing things began to happen! My instructor would regularly say things that felt like messages from the Universe reaching straight to my heart. When I was struggling and fighting the inevitable, I would learn to surrender. When I was guilt-tripping myself about not being perfect, I would learn not to force myself. Through my yoga practice I learned that I don't have to figure everything out, I just show up to the work and everything works itself out.

The discovery of yoga has been a tremendous blessing for me. Not only has it mediated my anxiety, it has made me a happier person and I feel more like I belong in the universe. It's given me a relationship with my body and my feelings and has helped me feel like a whole person rather than a bunch of jumbled parts. Most importantly, yoga has helped me to feel loved.

What more beautiful gift can we ask for than to feel and be loved? This is a divine rite for all of us and can be found by detaching from our fear and learning to trust our intuition.

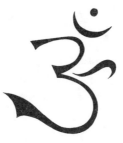

Chapter Nine

Empower Yourself with Balance

Yoga and balance are synonymous with each other. When we think of yoga, we can visualize standing on one leg, supporting our body with our hands, or even standing on our head without falling over. When we think of balance, we may also think of holding ourselves in stillness. Many of us feel it is something not easily achieved and is for a more advanced student. The truth is, balance is for everyone.

We need balance in our lives so that we may experience opposites. If we do not know suffering, then how can we know the full extent of joy? If we have never felt self-conscious, then how can we know the power of self-confidence? It is balance that allows us to experience the full extent of our emotions and our world by putting into perspective both sides of duality. Without it our world would be chaotic, with no equilibrium. In the words of Edgar Cayce, one of the world's most renowned "seers" and psychics, "Everything in moderation." Balance is the key. Especially in our dualistic world of night and day, black and white, male and female, dark and light, we must maintain a balance between the two extremes in order to find our center, our inner awareness.

As the *Bhagavad-Gita* states, yoga is balance. When we are balanced inwardly, we are able to balance our outward experiences to our environment. This means as we concentrate on our breath and body awareness through our yoga practice on the mat, we begin to live in balance with relationship to our job, our family, friends, and especially to ourselves.

Empowerment comes with this inner balance because when we approach life with a calm and centered attitude, we are able to survey each situation and act accordingly without having to react to unexpected and chaotic events. Even if we feel our outside circumstances are overwhelming, we can stay calm internally and weather the storm as it rages around us. Balance teaches us to listen to ourselves and to those around us, thus enabling us to act accordingly without having to blindly react to people and situations.

Dharana

Dharana is, in essence, asana applied to our mind. Its meaning is concentration and it is the sixth limb of Patanjali's eight-fold path. It consists of the uninterrupted focusing of attention on a single mental object, which leads to meditation. Concentration involves teaching our mind to focus on one thing at a time instead of many different things at once. Multitasking has become a very popular way of getting things accomplished in our society, which shows our increased sense of urgency and our lack of one-pointed focus. We may think that we are honing our concentration skills by thinking of many things at once, but in fact, we are diluting our focus and attention, thus not comprehending the deepest understanding of one single thing.

It is possible to stand on the sharpened edge of a knife, but it is difficult for an unprepared person to stand in the concentrations of Yoga.

—The Mahabharata, one of India's great epics which encompasses the *Bhagavad-Gita*

Dharana teaches us to concentrate on one thing, whether it is our mantra, our breath, a candle flame, or a blade of grass. By becoming adept at concentrating, we focus our attention more deeply on our higher Self and ultimately our Divine existence, which is God.

We can achieve this deep concentration spontaneously by softly opening to the experience rather than forcing attempts with mind control. Dharana is not about controlling the mind, but is regarded as opening our mind through one-pointed concentration. With the ability to concentrate fully on one object without the distractions of other thoughts, we are able to bring our mind to a quiet, centered place of balance, which prepares us to move into meditation. This place is where we are open to hearing the whispers of God, our higher Self.

To some, this concept may seem overwhelming due to the constant chattering of the mind. Don't let your full and active life deter you from experiencing focused concentration. More than anything else, practicing dharana will make your life flow more easily with its practice of concentration. When you can focus on one thing at a time, you will be able to achieve greater results with your actions and you will find deeper understanding of what you focus upon.

Beyond Mental Concentration

Our minds are like vast computer databases that can, at times, process information faster than we can comprehend it. Through study, research, and life lessons, we increase our knowledge and the amount of information stored in our minds. Having such a huge storehouse of information is quite helpful for experiencing our outside world, but what about experiencing our inner world? Is it possible that our mind can be oversaturated with information?

The world is a reflection of your mind. As your mind clears, you perceive reality simply as it is.
—Dan Millman, author of Way of the Peaceful Warrior

Perhaps the answer doesn't lie in reducing the amount of knowledge that we store in our minds but in how we store and use that knowledge. For example, I have a friend who is by far one of the most brilliant people I know. He is multi-talented and is really good at whatever he puts his mind to. I am not exaggerating here! This man seems to know about everything from wine to foreign languages, from science to outdoor survival and most everything in between. He gives his all to every project he undertakes and always accomplishes them in a first-rate manner. He continually amazes me.

For most of us, if we spread our attention in that many directions, we wouldn't know which end was up, much less be able to concentrate enough to do a good job on *any* of our projects. There comes a time when the mind must let go of all the tasks, chatter, and negative self-talk that it heaps upon itself in order to regroup and focus on what truly is important.

Now, back to my friend. It would appear that he has everything together and is quite focused. This may be true outwardly because his professional life is quite successful with a string of accomplishments. Upon a deeper look, however, his mind may have focused on his talents and tasks, but his concentration beyond the mind still needs some focus.

Even though he has accomplished many things, he can't seem to get out of the rut of "thinking." It's true we must concentrate to think and we must focus our concentration if we want to accomplish tasks. However, if we are to find our true Self and our reason for existence, we must move past the mind to a single-pointed focus that releases the mind chatter and distractions.

This concentration is what Patanjali refers to as dharana. When we hold our mind in a motionless state, placing our attention inward, not even aware of our outer surroundings, we achieve deeper concentration as a whole-body experience free from physical tension. It has an extraordinary dimension of mystical depth, in which inner creativity unfolds from higher consciousness. We regularly achieve this state while practicing yoga. As we move and breathe into each asana our focus is beyond the mind, resting upon the experience of each pose. Nothing else permeates this focus, and thus we can reach a true mind/body/spirit connection.

We've all experienced those moments when we've either said or done something and we were amazed at how we accomplished the outcome. Many times in the classes I teach, I find that what I say comes from somewhere beyond my mental thoughts. The wisdom comes through me from my higher Self and I am amazed at its profundity. Think back to the time you painted that beautiful picture of the ocean and were pleasantly surprised at how well it turned out considering you weren't even sure how to get started. Perhaps you made plans to create a magnificent garden and weren't quite sure how you were going to accomplish the task, only to see the results of your labor and stand in amazement of how it evolved. These are examples of taking our focus beyond mental concentration. When we surrender, letting go of our mental "to-do" lists, we are free to experience the concentration of higher consciousness.

Inner Balance

If we are unbalanced in any of our chakra energies, we may feel unstable, insecure, confused, and afraid. Instead of seeing a universe of abundance and joy, we may experience it as scarcity and fear. Being centered is the difference between reaching to the next level of awareness and getting swallowed in the chaos of unnecessary mind chatter. Without this internal equilibrium, we cannot be present for our daily activities and thus we will have difficulty experiencing joy and peace in our lives. This is why having inner balance is so important to achieving peace and stability in our outer world.

> If you are unable to find the truth right where you are, where else do you expect to find it?
> —Dogen (1200–1253), Buddhist priest

Yoga helps us balance our chakras and become more centered in our physical body. Through practice we become more connected to the earth, feeling grounded and strong like a tree that sends roots deep into the soil with branches reaching upward toward the sky to our higher awareness. As we connect our body with our mind, spirit begins to emerge, creating a conscious inner balance from which we can approach life.

A job change, the breakup of a relationship, a move, an argument, or other crises can affect our sense of being grounded and being centered. Even a positive life change, such as getting married or having a baby, can throw us off balance. Yoga helps us strengthen our foundation, increase our concentration, and connect our head—our mental world—with our body—the physical world—to integrate the full experience of a balanced life.

Although clearing mind chatter is important, inner balance is much more than that. It is essentially the attitude of looking at life for what it is, without being drastically affected by its ups and downs. This means that when we find ourselves caught in the middle of rush hour traffic, we are able to relax, realizing that we aren't going to go anywhere quickly and using our extra time to practice deep yogic breathing. If we go with the flow of life, we can achieve internal as well as external balance. When we resist life as it is, we lose our inner balance and the ability to make clear and honest decisions. We even lose the freedom of being still.

It isn't always easy holding on to the inner balance that we seek; that is why a yoga practice is essential to bringing us back to that state of equanimity. Keep in mind that a centered yoga practice doesn't have to stay on your mat. Whenever you find yourself getting upset or losing your equilibrium, begin to consciously breathe. Fill your lungs completely and become aware of the length of your inhalations and exhalations. Once your breathing becomes more relaxed and focused, then try standing in Mountain Pose (see Chapter 1) or folding into a forward bend. These postures help ground you and calm your nerves. They allow you to focus your mind and relax into that centered, calm place within from where you are the viewer of your life instead of the actor. From here you can not only see balance unfolding, but you can feel it.

London Bridge Is Falling Down

Can you remember being a child and playing London Bridge with your friends? Two children would hold each other's hands above their heads, making a bridge for the rest of the kids to walk under while everyone sang "London bridge is falling down, falling down ...." When we sang the phrase "my fair lady," the two kids holding hands would drop their arms around one child, trapping her and shaking her around before they would release her to freedom. With that, we'd start all over again singing London Bridge and circling under the bridge, this time with the trapped child becoming part of the bridge.

> Only let the moving waters calm down, and the sun and moon will be reflected on the surface of your being.
>
> —Rumi, poet

I use this analogy to explain how it sometimes feels when life seems to crash all around us and we feel trapped and unable to help ourselves. We may be dealing with such intense challenges as a life-threatening illness, losing our job, or surviving a divorce. We may even be stressed with less severe events such as making our way through rush hour traffic, organizing the company Christmas party, or putting the kids to bed when they don't want to go. Regardless of the severity of the challenge, it is during these times when we must gather ourselves together, reach deep inside, and find the balance that is within us.

One important and empowering way to find our balance is through yoga. When we practice, we are making the commitment to concentrate on ourselves, on our health, on our breathing. We release outside distractions and focus only on the present moment. Through this concentration, we acknowledge to ourselves and state to those around us that we are important and that we are worthy to have radiant health, abundant love, and fulfilling relationships with others as well as with ourselves. This statement does not mean that we are better than others, but that we are equally important and we recognize this fact. Through this inner personal work, we fortify ourselves to meet the challenges of our life with calm resolve, or at least with understanding and less stress. With a regular yoga practice of forward and backward bends, along with twists and balancing poses, we can handle when "the London Bridge" falls down around us.

Practice: Gazing

The meditative practice of gazing has a Sanskrit term called *tratak*, sometimes referred to as *trataka*. It refers to the steady, relaxed gazing at a flame (or any object except for the sun) until tears begin to fill the eyes. In the yogic texts it is said to cure diseases of the eyes and also increase clairvoyance.

I could see forever as I gazed into your eyes and all of a sudden forever was all there was …

—Bliss Wood, author and yoga instructor

This practice can greatly improve our ability to focus. Although using a flame to concentrate on is ideal, we can choose any object to fix our gaze on to bring about this one-pointed focus. A flower, a tree, a picture of someone dear, and even a spot on the wall can be used to achieve our goal. The only object that we should never gaze upon is the sun, due to its intense light, which can damage our eyes and even cause blindness.

Try this practice on your own either before meditation or by itself. To begin, it only takes about one to three minutes, and you can extend the time as your eyes adjust. It is not uncommon to achieve profound benefits with the practice of tratak.

Make sure you are in a comfortable seated position. Place a candle about arm's length away from you at eye level so that you can sit up tall, looking straight ahead. Gaze at the flame without blinking for between one and three minutes, until your eyes begin to water and tears roll down your cheeks. This process cleanses your eyes and your tear ducts. Once your eyes start to water, close them and concentrate on the shadow image of the flame that is in your mind's eye. Try keeping your closed lid gaze between your eyes as you focus on the alter-image of the flame. What do you see? What color is the image in your mind? How does this exercise make you feel emotionally?

If you used tratak as a preliminary to meditation, notice if there were any significant changes to that. Were you able to sit in meditation for a longer period of time, going deeper into awareness? Did you find your meditation to be more interactive with your intuition? These are just some of the situations that might occur. Pay attention to how you feel and what comes to you while you are meditating. For the sake of clarity, write down your experiences either after you finish the practice of tratak or when you finish your meditation, and then re-read what you have written.

This practice can profoundly deepen your yoga and meditation practices by placing your concentration on your higher Self, which is a deeper focus than even gathering your mental thoughts. It also improves our eyesight, which can be most helpful when we are fatigued and stressed. When I have finished tratak, I find that my whole being is much more relaxed, less reactionary, and able to make choices that empower me rather than cause me to lose my focus.

Experiment with this practice of gazing and watch how it gathers all the fragmented pieces of your being back to your Self. Find out for yourself how empowering it is to have such concentration that you even catch a glimpse of who you really are and why you are here on this earth!

Concentrated Physical Balance

We've been talking a lot about mental focus and emotional balance, so now it's only appropriate that we address our physical balance. For many of us, this can mean quite the challenge when it comes to yoga postures. Although yoga offers many postures that are relaxing and increase our flexibility, it is known for its ability to bring strength and balance into the life of the practitioner.

Most balancing postures require physical strength in order to achieve the full extent of the pose, and many of us tend to shy away from these magnificent and empowering asanas because we don't feel we have the strength to hold such a powerful pose. The truth is that balancing postures are imperative to a well-rounded practice and a calmer, more balanced life.

There are many variations for the beginner to try which don't feel as difficult to hold physically. These variations empower our mental and emotional bodies, which then supports our physical body. Can you see how beautifully our mind, our emotions, and our physical body work together to create the whole that is us?

Here is an example of how one of my students, David, has become aware of and achieved greater balance through the practice of yoga. This is just one example of how important physical balance is to us:

Within the last several years I have taken up rock climbing as part of my participation with the Boy Scouts. The scouts in my troop enjoy climbing and rappelling, so this activity requires trained adult leadership. Once I was trained for the scouts, my interest in climbing increased and I have been climbing frequently ever since. Within the last few months, I began taking yoga to improve my balance and flexibility and I have found, through my participation in yoga, that I am able to balance over my feet better which saves my strength for climbing. At the same time, the stretching positions have increased my flexibility, which allows me to reach the holds easier and stay closer to the climbing surface. Yoga has made me a safer and more balanced climber and has returned some flexibility from my younger days.

As you can see from David's story, not only did his physical balance improve, but through the physical improvement he gained confidence and mental concentration. His yoga classes enabled him to experience his life in a much more adventurous and fulfilling way.

Think of something in your life that requires you to have physical balance. Is balance easy for you or difficult? Does your physical balance affect your mental concentration and your emotional stability? These questions are posed just to bring your awareness back to your center, so be honest with yourself. When we know what we need to work on and we focus our intent, we can then accomplish great things in a short amount of time. Would you like to improve your total balance? If so, get to your mat, focus on your breath, and let your body stand on its own two feet.

One-Pointed Focus

Can you remember a time in your life when you were so focused on something that you weren't aware of anything else around you? Perhaps you were sketching the clouds on a crisp autumn day, putting together your child's new swing set, completing your taxes for the end of the quarter, or practicing a series of yoga postures. In any case, did you notice how time seemed to fly when you finally finished your project even though it felt like a short time? These are all examples of one-pointed focus. Your concentration was so complete that no outside distractions could affect you.

One-pointed focus in the context of dharana is a firm and steady attention upon a particular internal object within the body. This concept takes our concentration one step further from mental focus on an object outside of ourselves. The Bhagavad-Gita states that to find true happiness and peace we need to release the clutter of our mind and be still. When we can relax into a state of stillness, focusing on our breath, a mantra, or our higher Self, we are able to free ourselves from outside distractions. This concentration is what motivates our creativity and deepens our wisdom. It makes us aware of our motivations so we can clearly see our actions and reactions in our daily life.

When we are mindful within, we can be more conscious with our actions and words in our outer world. This is precisely why the practice of yoga is paramount in reducing stress and increasing concentration in our life. While we are on our mat, we focus on breathing, turn our awareness inward, and practice the mindful movements of asana. These actions bring us to that one-pointed focus in which we come to know the empowered nature of our true and highest Self.

Natarajasana (Dancing Shiva Pose)

Nataraja (Lord of Dance) is another name for Shiva, the Hindu god who is the destroyer of our delusions and illusions. He symbolizes our inner force that uncovers and destroys our short-sighted, created concepts of the world, so that we may let go of our illusions and see reality, life as it truly is.

Not everyone will accept Shiva as a deity or even an historical figure; however, we can apply the lessons of this story to our own lives. If, through balancing our inner awareness, we can let go of the illusions of fear and self-consciousness in our lives, we can then see the reality of who we really are. We are not our career, nor are we the perceptions that we hold of ourselves. We are pure consciousness that is creative and boundless in nature. We have unlimited potential born from all possibilities.

Practicing Natarajasana helps us to see and feel our pure potential through the balancing effects it creates in our body. The movement of this pose comes from our center and extends outward in all directions. It requires foundational strength as well as flexibility in our legs. In reaching forward though our chest and leading arm and lengthening back into the lifted leg, we are opening the front side of our body and our heart into an expansive acceptance of the present moment.

When we find balance in this pose, there is nothing else but one-pointed concentration through the interaction between body and mind. Our body supports the concentration of the mind by focusing our awareness in the present moment of physical balance. Likewise, the mind's inner balance allows the body to surrender into a state of equilibrium.

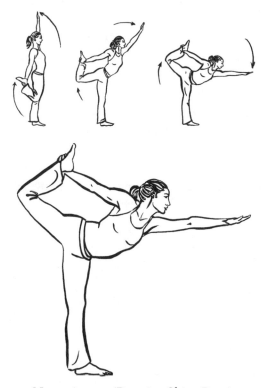

Natarajasana (Dancing Shiva Pose).

Empowerment Exercise: Natarajasana

Natarajasana Affirmation: *I am empowered through the balance of my body, mind, and emotions.*

Natarajasana is an excellent example of using our mind and body to create focused concentration. Through this focus, we feel empowered in the pose and can then take this feeling into our daily lives to enrich and empower our relationships with our Self and with others:

1. Stand in Tadasana (Mountain Pose, see Chapter 1). Inhale, shift your weight onto your right foot, and lift your left heel toward your left buttock as you bend the knee.

2. Rotate your left shoulder outward, turning the palm of your hand outward, and drop your left hand down to the inside of your left ankle and hold it.

3. Bring both knees together, extending through the right leg and pressing the pelvic girdle forward while dropping your tailbone toward the floor. Continue lifting upward through your solar plexus.

4. Raise your right arm straight over your head, keeping your arm slightly behind your ear. (Beginners may stay in this position. It is a simplified version of Natarajasana called Stork Pose.)

5. Inhale, extend upward through the torso and right arm as you ground down into your standing leg.

6. Exhale, in unison (keeping the stretch even) lift your left foot up, away from the floor and back, away from your buttocks. Extend your left thigh behind you and parallel to the floor. Reach your right arm forward, keeping your chest lifted, and bring your arm parallel to the floor.

7. Breathe evenly through the pose for as long as you can balance. Begin with five to eight rounds of breath and work your way to at least one minute.

8. Repeat to the other side for the same length of time.

Benefits

This posture is one of my most favorite balancing poses. It may look difficult to do but don't let that deter you from experiencing the benefits of this wonderful asana. As stated in the previous instructions, you may begin by practicing its variation of Stork Pose.

Improved balance is one of the main reasons for doing Natarajasana; however, it is not the only benefit to this empowering pose. It strengthens our legs and ankles, enhancing our first chakra and enabling us to feel grounded and secure in our bodies. It also stretches our thighs, groin, and abdomen, which stimulates our second and third chakras. In stretching and opening up our pelvic girdle, we can stimulate creativity through our second chakra. As we lift through the posture and stretch our solar plexus, we stimulate our third chakra and thus strengthen our resolve and self-confidence.

Natarajasana stretches the shoulders and chest, which on the physical level creates more space for the lungs to expand. When the lungs have more room to move, your breath can grow deeper and fuller, thus being more satisfying. Stretching through the chest and heart center, your fourth chakra also stimulates emotional feelings and responses, triggered through cellular memory.

If you find that you experience some emotional feeling or memory, breathe into it and ground more deeply into your standing leg for balance. Not only will you feel empowered for having accomplished such a beautiful balancing posture, you will experience the satisfaction of balancing through emotional releases.

Find your inner strength in your ability to balance physically, emotionally, and mentally during your yoga practice. Then take that balance and expand it into your daily life by thinking before you react to situations, experiencing your emotions as the observer, even if they are uncomfortable, without getting swept away either with mania or depression.

Balancing postures help you to take control and stop blaming outside circumstances for your life. This realization is more powerful than any excuse you could ever think up and will fill your life with abundance, grace, and empowerment.

Cautions

When attempting Natarajasana, there are a few things to consider. If you have high or low blood pressure, it is wise to practice the Stork Pose variation throughout your practice. Check with your doctor regarding your blood pressure to make sure it is manageable before attempting the full extent of this pose. (Regular practice of Ujjayi Breath and Savasana have been known to relieve high blood pressure.)

You may also want to consider your lower back and knees in this posture as it requires much strength and stretching through these areas. If you have serious lower back and/or knee problems, do not attempt to come to Natajarasana without first warming up for some time and checking with your doctor.

As with any posture, use your intuition and trust the feelings of your body. Never push yourself into a pose; rather, play your edge and ease into each asana.

Real Life

The following the story is of how Brendi found yoga. In a sense, her situation shows surrender in the way she finally let go of opinions of others and old ways of thinking, which then gave her the opportunity to find new possibilities and a healthier way to live. Through surrender, Brendi was able to find balance in her body and in her life, which has led to a more focused concentration of what truly works in her life and what doesn't.

"My first experience with yoga was for a work assignment. I was to familiarize myself with all the exercise programs offered at my workplace. In return, when I met with clients I could advise them on which programs might best fit them.

I was a long-time jogger and had been working with free weights for some time. I had recently experienced some neurological problems and was having weakness in my right hand and leg, difficulty with coordination in my right arm and hand, numbness in both my arms, and back/hip pain.

I had been to several physicians and had multiple tests done. The conclusion was that my symptoms were either related to two bulging disks in my spine or that I might be experiencing the first signs of multiple sclerosis. I was terrified. The doctor prescribed physical therapy and asked me to stop jogging. The physical therapy gave me little results and a lot of frustration. The exercises they gave me were too easy, the cost was ridiculous, and the therapist didn't have enough time to spend with me.

I was feeling anxiety not only from my illness but also from not being able to do my regular workout. I decided to stop physical therapy and work with a personal trainer to help build my strength back. Over time my symptoms improved, but did not go away.

As instructed by my boss, I went to one of the yoga classes at our facility. At the beginning it was very uncomfortable for me because it made me aware of all my symptoms. However, after the first class, I realized for the first time in many months my back and hip pain was gone. It only lasted for a few hours but after each class I took, the pain was gone. After several months of classes, my back pain was nonexistent and so were my other symptoms.

Although I was thrilled to have my symptoms relieved, even more exciting for me was to find an exercise that relaxed my mind. After all my years of jogging and other types of exercise, I had never found anything that could stop my mind from thinking. While I would be working out my mind would wander; what should I do about my work problem, my kids problems, what do I need to get done today, where did I leave my watch, etc. …. Yoga freed my mind …. *No thinking* … what a gift! I found that when I walked out of my yoga class my stress was lowered and I had a great workout. One whole hour of a peaceful mind!

As I continued with my weekly yoga classes, the instructor showed us many postures which challenged my balance and my ability to stay in my center. One of my favorite balancing poses is Dancing Shiva Pose (Natarajasana). When I first began to work on this pose I was unable to do it with any luck at all. When I was having my worst episodes of weakness I had difficulty with any type of balance. This pose became my gauge of return to wellness. Each week my progress inched forward as I could hold the posture a couple more seconds. Each second was a step toward total recovery. When I finally was able to hold my pose for 30 seconds I felt I had reached my goal. This continues to be one of my favorite poses reminding me to be grateful for my health and strength."

Empowerment Journal

This chapter has focused primarily on balance, both internal and physical. We have witnessed through Brendi's real-life story how particular postures affect our physical balance as well as creating a calm center. Balance, however, is much more than holding a physical posture or clearing our mind from unwanted clutter. It is a combination of the two, gracefully performed throughout our daily life.

There are only three things you need to let go of: judging, controlling, and being right. Release these three and you will have the whole mind and twinkly heart of a child.

—Hugh Prather, author

The following journal entry comes from a very good friend of mine who is a prominent figure in promoting the mind/body/spirit movement throughout the health-care field. Carrie's comments regarding how yoga has personally brought balance to her life show how internal concentration and focus can dramatically change life in the external world. Her comments (as well as her life) clearly depict a dramatic shift of awareness from external resistance, forcing, and tension to balance through self-love, acceptance, and empowered living:

Yoga has had a dramatic impact on my life. It has been instrumental in my healing process. First and foremost, it has helped me fall in love with myself, unconditionally.

For years I was a disciplined exerciser. I kept my body in tip-top shape. Unfortunately, I approached exercise as a form of self-punishment. I never really saw myself as "good enough." I felt I was not thin enough, fit enough, or even pretty enough. I thought, to be someone, I had to look like the models in the magazines. I had cut off my body from my mind and my spirit. I had lost the balance of a fully empowered human being.

Through yoga I began to "sew my head back onto my body." I began to pay attention to the subtle messages my body was sending me. I started to appreciate and love my body. This helped me to slow down and to connect with God, my personal values, and other people. I am constantly amazed at how yoga enables me to feel energized and grounded all at the same time. Yoga has touched every aspect of my life, giving balance to my inner life as well as my outside world.

I can now say that I am a healthy, strong, and empowered woman. Through the practice of yoga I have found a centered calm, a balance like I've never known before. I can't imagine my life without this wonderful spirit/mind/body "work-in," called yoga.

Mantras for Daily Living

You may find that use of a mantra makes it easier to practice yoga asanas that are particularly difficult, like balancing postures or inversions. As you balance in the pose, recite your mantra either silently, whispered, or out loud and watch how you become steadier in your pose.

As you complete your yoga practice, take your mantra with you into your day and recite it whenever you feel you are losing your mental balance. A mantra is an instrument of conscious intention, used for empowerment. It can reinforce the work you do on the mat so that it enhances the way you live your life. Also, it will reinforce the physical memories of the work you accomplished on your mat as it associates the physical with the sound of the mantra.

For example, if you practice the balancing asana of Vrkasana (Tree Pose) and repeat the mantra "I am calm and centered" while you are holding the pose, the mantra will automatically trigger the physical responses in your body. This is true when you recite it at any time during the day, even after you've completed the pose. This is how your mantra continues to support you throughout your daily routines. Mantras are part of what enables us to take our yoga from the mat and into our life.

Here are some examples for you to consider. As always, however, find or create a mantra that resonates with you. This will help to deepen your practice, making its effects more powerful in your life.

- "Stability gives me wings to fly."
- "I am balanced in love, peace, and light."
- "I am grateful for the joy of being me."
- "Open heart. Open mind. Balanced freedom."
- "My life is balanced. I am free."
- "I love life."
- "I am calm and centered."

Finding Balance in Surrender

When we first think of the word "surrender," most likely we associate it with defeat and disempowerment. From our ego's point of view, this is a totally rational understanding. However, from a spiritual insight, surrender is finding balance between our desires and reality. It is being open to receive whatever comes to us. In that openness, we can make conscious choices and have clear understandings of what will truly support us in our lives. There is no attachment to illusion or controlling of the outcome of a situation. Surrender is complete acceptance of what is and the ability to be of service without attachment.

Spiritually, no action is more important than surrender.
—Deepak Chopra, best-selling author and physician

As we practice yoga and move through each asana, we find a balance between pushing our edge and surrendering into relaxation. If we ignore our boundaries and push too far because of ego, we risk injuring ourselves and balance eludes us. On the other hand, if we shy away from finding our edge, the point of our growth, we still do not achieve balance because we have not stretched our awareness far enough to know our limits. Balance arrives at the point in which we meet our resistance and surrender into it.

When we surrender to what is, we have no need to oppose reality. Our feelings are more important than results of our actions, and we desire to be of service to others. When we are balanced through the act of surrendering our ego, we achieve a state of oneness with all beings. It becomes easy to see how we are connected to our spouse, our children, our friends, and even our pets because we have taken the separate "I" out of our consciousness by letting go of our need to be special. Through surrendering we realize that we are all equal, none more special than another. Equanimity can permeate our senses when we release our need to be separate. Once that happens we find empowerment through inner balance and one-pointed concentration, which leads us further into our exploration of our true Self.

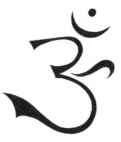

Chapter Ten

Moving Into Stillness

Every day, in the silence of dawn, before the birds begin to chirp, before the sun peeks over the horizon, before the world begins to stir, there is a moment of complete and utter stillness. This moment is our glimpse into the vast awareness of our Spirit.

Yoga can bring this same stillness to us each time we practice. Our full concentration rests in our centered awareness as we move from one posture to the next. As we settle into the movement of our body and breath, the mind chatter begins to diminish and our concentration naturally leads us into a meditative state where we become conscious of ourselves, experiencing the present moment. In this state of meditation, we have entered a peaceful and calm emotional equilibrium accompanied by an awareness that is greater than when we are awake. We have let go of our external environment and entered into the empowered state of meditation.

Can you think of a time when you experienced stillness, whether you were drifting off to sleep, gazing into the eyes of your newborn child, sitting in meditation, or strolling through the woods for your morning walk? Did you notice an expanded sense of yourself or a more peaceful feeling than normal?

Perhaps you received spontaneous answers to the questions that had been on your mind. When we become still internally and listen to the subtle communications of our body, mind, and emotions, we are able to tap into that all-knowing place of higher consciousness, of God.

Dhyana

Dhyana is the seventh limb of the Yoga Sutras and is referred to as the state of meditative absorption where we no longer mentally concentrate on an object, but we experience it with complete awareness in a calm and peaceful state. When we reach the state of dhyana, we are no longer attached to the object of our focus; we become one with the object of focus.

The paradox of meditation is that it both empties the mind and, at the same time, encourages alertness.
—John H. Clark, British psychologist

Think of a time when you took a walk in a beautiful area and you noticed the trees, the sky above, all the animals and birds and the earth below. You experienced your walk with all five of your physical senses, relishing the sights, sounds, smells, textures, and perhaps even the taste of your surroundings. Even though you may have stopped occasionally to touch a fallen leaf or to dip your fingers in the babbling brook, you did not linger too long in one place. You kept walking, absorbing nature's encompassing beauty, attaching to nothing but experiencing everything.

It is the same with dhyana. We experience the full spectrum of awareness in meditation, yet we do not attach ourselves to the object we are meditating on. It's as if we become one with what we are focused on. The observer and the observed are one in the same. We trust that our higher Self is the Experiencer of all.

When we can perceive ourselves as being one with all of creation, we can then understand compassion and feel the connection with all beings. As we begin to feel more connected, our lives become more of a living meditation. In everything we do we have more awareness. It makes it easier for us to think before we speak or take action. We are more prone to a calm and peaceful disposition, and especially, we experience our lives from an empowered state of consciousness. Self-confidence and humility are strong characteristics of someone who meditates.

Dhyana, or meditative absorption, grows out of dharana, a prolonged and deepened concentration. Naturally, it is the next step from having one-pointed focus to being the one-pointed focus.

Meditation

Meditation is more than a practice or a religious rite that we must be initiated into. It is a universal phenomenon that encompasses much more than sitting on a cushion chanting "Om," or putting our bodies in difficult and sometimes painful contortions. Meditation is merely a device to make us aware of our real Self. It is so simple and yet can most profoundly empower our life. Just as the sun and moon light our outer world, meditation illuminates our inner world. Its essence is the art of being aware of what is going on inside as well as around us.

Don't just do something ... sit there!
—Anonymous

This awareness has been said to be the greatest adventure that our mind can undertake. It is the perfect act of "being." When we are in a state of being, there is no action, no thought, no emotional stirring. We just are and in that state, we become the witness to our pure, joyful Self. This concept is so simple, yet the thought of being a witness to our own Self gets a little confusing until we actually experience withdrawing our awareness from everywhere and just let it rest within ourselves.

So then, how do we meditate? How do we get to the point where we let go of all our outside responsibilities and obligations? How do we turn inward and leave the outside world behind? Keep in mind, meditation is not about escaping from our life and responsibilities, nor is it a supernatural practice that makes us better than anyone else. Rather, it unifies us with everything and everyone, and this empowers our very existence.

The first step of this meditative awareness is in watching our body. Slowly we become alert to our breath, our gestures, movements, and where we hold our tension. The more alert we are to these bodily sensations, the more relaxed and attuned we become. A sense of peace begins to envelop us.

The next part of meditation is in becoming aware of our thoughts. They are subtler than our body so it may take a little more time to achieve this awareness. Once we realize how our thoughts affect our life we can see the insane chattering that is not based in reality which throws us out of our center. The release of the negative mind chatter is part of what we achieve through meditation.

As our attention settles deeper into our body and mind we can then bring our awareness to our emotions, reflecting on our moods and feelings. When this unity between body, mind, and emotions is present, we can feel a sense of oneness within ourselves which expands our awareness even further to the awakened state of perfect stillness. In this stillness, we now come to know supreme happiness and bliss.

The basic thought is that meditation can only be practiced while sitting still, and this has scared many people away from the empowering benefits that it can bring. Meditation can be practiced anywhere and through any action as long as we are observing the action. It is the quality of the observation that is important, not the action itself. So when we are out for our daily jog, we can meditate on the movement of our legs, our arms, our breath without concentrating on the act of jogging. Likewise, when we are cooking a meal for our family we can meditate on how we combine and prepare the foods for each dish without thinking of the actual meal.

Meditation is watching, and therefore we become alert to the act of watching rather than the finished product of our efforts. In the same manner, we can meditate in stillness, becoming the watcher of our bodily sensations, our thoughts, and our emotions until even the awareness of watching merges into an awakened state of ultimate joy.

Obstacles to Meditation

Many people give me reasons why they think meditation won't fit into their lives. In fact, I've struggled at times with my own internal dialogue giving me excuses as to why I don't have enough time to meditate. Even now, after meditating for many years, my mind will come up with excuses for not taking the time to sit and be open to all possibilities.

There are only two difficulties on the path of meditation: one is the ego and the other is your constantly chattering mind.
—Osho, existentialist and spiritual leader from India

I find great peace and clarity with meditation and always feel better after I have taken the time to either sit on my cushion or meditatively walk through the woods. So why, then, does my mind make excuses?

As Osho states in the previous quote, the ego and a constantly chattering mind are the two obstacles to meditation. All other challenges stem from these two concepts. Meditation, through relaxed, clear witnessing, is an empowerment tool because it allows us to see our connection with everything. Through meditation we know that we are connected to the earth and everything on it. We can feel the unity through our breath. Every time we breathe in oxygen we are connecting with the trees and plants that produce it. In turn, as we exhale, we are giving back to them the carbon dioxide that they need to sustain life. There is a bridge that connects all of existence.

Can you think of other examples of how you are connected to the whole of this earth? Think of how another person makes you feel love, joy, and happiness. What are the qualities that you connect with in that person? On the other hand, think of someone (or something) that makes you feel sad, unhappy, or frustrated and angry. Even though these emotions are not pleasant, you are still connected to this person (or thing) because of the feelings and thoughts you share. If we were not connected, then we would not feel anything from another. We would not be affected by someone else's story.

The ego sees itself as separate from the world and from each other, which causes a struggle. From this separateness comes competition, fear, and struggle. It's not necessarily that our ego is bad, because its ultimate goal is to protect us. However, modern society and psychology has educated us to believe that the stronger our ego, the more successful we will be in our professional lives as well as our personal lives. We've been taught that a strong and healthy ego produces assertiveness.

The danger in this way of thinking is that it causes separateness. Our ego thinks in terms of "me" and "mine" versus "you" and "yours." As we think in this manner, we introduce such feelings as insecurity, fear of rejection, judgment, and narcissism. Our sense of peace, oneness, and connection has been lost, which in turn makes us search outside of ourselves for remedies to ease our pain and fear.

As we mask our pain with the accumulation of material things, power, politics, and money, it makes it difficult to relax into a state of being without doing. Our mind chatter constantly reminds us of what we don't have and what is wrong with us. It fills our mind so there is no room to listen and to receive clarity and understanding.

This is how we run into difficulty with meditation. Once we make the commitment to relax our mind and let go of expectations, thoughts, and judgments, the ego and mind chatter will begin to thwart our intentions. We are, however, wiser than our ego and if we do not attach to our chattering mind, it will eventually surrender so that we settle into the stillness of meditation where we gain insight, peace, and higher awareness.

It is important not to judge yourself when you come to your meditation. Thoughts will inevitably come to your mind as you try to settle it. It is also possible that you will fall asleep as you sit quietly. The point we are trying to reach is the stillness of the "gap" between our thoughts. As we accept our meditation for what is, at any given moment, we surrender more deeply to the experience. Meditation takes practice, and it is best to start with just a minute or two of stillness and work up to five, ten, fifteen, even thirty minutes as your mind adjusts to the surrendering process. Most importantly, know that through your meditations you can transform mind chatter and your ego to create deep inner peace and serenity, which translates to an empowered and centered life.

Listen to Your Thoughts

The purpose of yogic meditation is to intercept the chatter of ordinary mental activity. Through this quieting of the mind we are able to listen more closely to what our thoughts are actually saying. It is also possible to hear guidance from our higher Self once we have let go of the needless mind chatter that so readily fills our brain.

Be still and know that I am God.
—The Holy Bible, Psalms 46:10

It isn't easy to always be aware of our internal dialogue. When our daily life gets hectic and it seems we have many different issues to think about, it's hard to distinguish the empowering, loving thoughts from the critical, self-doubting words that our mind can interject. It's as if we are moving in a fog, hearing voices but not being able to see their source; therefore, we move blindly in the direction of the voice we think we can hear. Sometimes this means that we gravitate toward negative self-talk or critical judgments of ourselves and others.

Yoga and meditation are the keys to clearing the fog in our brain and showing the source of all our thoughts. As we move into stillness and observe our thoughts, we can distinguish what empowers us and what causes pain. The negative talk stems from fear and has no basis in truth. When we listen to our thoughts and settle into meditation, we can accept the positive and empowering things we say more easily. It is even possible to transform our negative thoughts into positive ones.

Have you caught yourself saying something like "that was stupid," "you're such a dummy," or "you're ugly" to yourself? Things like "I'm too fat," "I'm too short," "I'm not good enough" all indicate to our sub-conscious mind that we are not worthy and therefore we feel judged and rejected. Unfortunately, we have done all of this to ourselves because of some high standard our society has set. The bombardment of constant advertising for better bodies, beautiful skin, stronger muscles, and more money and power all filter into our self-talk.

By paying attention to what we hear, we can choose what we tell ourselves. Becoming still enough to distinguish the positive from the negative thoughts is imperative, and we do this through meditation. When we listen to our thoughts more consciously, we fortify ourselves with positive internal feedback and we empower our life through the loving thoughts that we think.

Practice: Placing Intentions

Prayer is referred to as talking to God, while meditation is said to be listening to God. Paying attention to what we say in prayer as well as how we use words in our everyday language can make the difference in how we manifest our intentions. For example, the phrase "I want ..." seems like a good way to ask for what we want; however, our subconscious mind is hearing that we are in a state of want and it will manifest this state of wanting for us.

Self-trust is the first secret to success.

—Ralph Waldo Emerson, American essayist and philosopher

Most of our prayers are either asking for something or giving thanks for what we have already received. Our subconscious mind is not subjective, nor is the Universe, our higher Self, so when we ask for something that we do not have, we are stating our lack. When we can give thanks for our intention, even before we have manifested the outcome, we are stating that we have what we desire.

Positive words such as love, happiness, thankfulness, joy, and peace fill our mind with contentment and greater awareness, while words like hate, can't, no, and don't give the signal to our brain of negativity. This in turn closes off our awareness and puts us in a state of lack. Taking our prayer a step further, positive actions enforce our positive intentions.

For example, one of my most recent intentions was to get some help putting insulation in my attic. (I know this sounds very materialistic, but it just shows that all intentions are heard when we are conscious of how we ask for them.) One Sunday morning, before I met my friends at our usual brunch spot, I was up practicing my morning yoga postures and visualizing the insulation already in my attic. I felt its warmth throughout the house and was thankful that I had the insulation in my attic. As I sat down to meditate after yoga, my first thought was thankfulness for the insulation, then I shifted my attention to my sixth chakra, focused on my breathing, and began my mantra meditation. That was it. I didn't wonder how it would get accomplished and I didn't worry if I could pay for the help and materials. In short, I didn't give it another thought.

Later that morning while at brunch with my friends I mentioned that I was going to insulate my attic. With that one comment, two of my friends volunteered to help me and we set a date then and there. This is one small example of how powerful placing an intention can be. It is important to know what you want to manifest, to focus on it, and then let go after you have made your request.

Let's practice placing positive intentions. Taking about 10 minutes in the morning is best, but whenever you can find the time will work. Think about something that you would like to have in your life. See it clearly in your mind's eye, noticing the color, texture, any sounds or aromas, and see yourself with this object. Visualize yourself happy and content, fully enjoying what you have manifested. You may even want to write down in full detail what you are intending.

Once you have a clear picture in your mind, practice a yoga posture or two and as you move through the poses think about your intention and associate it with how your body feels in the yoga postures. As you breathe in feel your intention coming to you, and as you exhale send your intention outward to the Universe, God, as a prayer of thanksgiving for already having what you desire.

Now, meditate for as long as you feel comfortable. Say thank you for your manifested intention at the beginning of your meditation and then do not dwell on your intention anymore. Go about your life and then witness how your desire unfolds. It is important not to have any expectations of how, when, and where you will receive what you want. Remember, everything happens in its own time and of its own accord. Trust that it is so and be grateful for what you receive.

Perfection in Stillness

Stillness is about being fully in the moment, in total harmony with yourself and with the world around you. When you're on the mat, yoga helps you find a place of balance and stillness within. As you learn this lesson in your body when you practice the postures and breathing exercises, your body memorizes the feeling. The more you practice feeling this, the more aware you become of feelings of tension and stress. As you learn to observe your own reactions, you begin to realize that you always have a choice in every situation. You may not be able to change the outward situation, but you can choose how you will react to it. Practicing stillness gives you a quiet center from which to observe outward activity.

Yoga is a way of moving into stillness in order to experience the truth of who you are.
—Eric Schiffman, yoga instructor

We are energetic beings. Yoga teaches that we can make choices about what we do with the energies available to us. Practicing stillness allows energy to flow without blocks, tension, or restriction. The energy of the life force (known as prana; see Chapter 7) is always available. Yoga helps you move beyond the blocks, resistance, and inner conflicts that restrict the flow of energy through you. Breathing and postures teach your body to become a clearer conduit for the energy. Meditation teaches you how to still the chatter of monkey mind (those thoughts that distract and demand with constant inner noise) and become an open channel for this abundant life force.

Stillness is the power of being totally here and now, in the moment, with your entire being. You carry this stillness within your heart. When you are not wholeheartedly in the moment, you tend to be distracted, wanting to be in more than one place at a time. Stillness comes when you give undivided attention to what "is," allowing you to experience an exquisite deep peace that helps you relax inside and move into harmony with your heart.

Becoming still allows you to experience the life force moving through you and to tap into the essence of your own being. When you are in a place of stillness, everything becomes clear and you gain a more detached and higher perspective on whatever situation you are experiencing in this moment. As muddy water in a glass settles and clears with patient waiting, so your mind and emotions can settle and clarify when you choose to practice inner stillness. By choosing to focus on the moment with quiet awareness, you are more able to respond appropriately and make fully conscious choices instead of allowing yourself to be driven by unconscious forces. Practicing stillness prepares you to pay attention and observe your own life.

As you become more clear and quiet inside during your yoga and meditation practice, you'll become more and more able to take that stillness and inner certainty into your daily life. Though you may be sitting in a traffic jam, you can choose to practice the stillness and serenity of a lakeside sunset within your mind. Though the day is filled with many tasks, you can find clarity and peace as you focus on one task at a time, one moment at a time. Take a break for some yogic breathing at your desk. Stand in Tadasana (Mountain Pose; see Chapter 1) in line at the grocery store. Quiet your heart in stillness and remember who you are.

The Practice of Introspection

Introspection is fundamental to the practice of meditation and is key to creating stillness within. When we take the time to contemplate the events of our day, the words someone said to us, or even the words we said to someone else, we are stepping back out of the mainstream of our life and looking deeper into the meaning of our thoughts, words, and actions. We can then see how they affect us and how we have affected our surroundings.

Be silent, meditate and then peacefully go where your spirit guides you.
—Liz Hengber, songwriter

The more conscious we become of our motivations and the content of our thoughts, the more empowered we are to live our lives in truth without the illusion of fear and judgment. Meditation and yoga are two important ways of practicing introspection.

Through the stillness of meditation we become the witness of ourselves, seeing all of our weaknesses and strengths. We do not judge ourselves as we look inward, but we notice our thoughts and intentions. Through introspection we know what is right and what is wrong for us. We are able to trust our intuition and our gut feelings as to what direction we must take in order to accomplish our spiritual goals.

Yoga is another benefit, which heightens the practice of introspection. Using the movements of the postures and the physical feelings they create, we become more aware of how our body talks to us. Ask yourself an important question and become aware of how your body responds. Does your finger twitch? Do you feel a flutter in your stomach? Perhaps you experience a tension or relaxation in your neck. All of these responses are your body giving answers to the things you are pondering.

Try turning off the radio, television, and stereo for a while. Don't even read a book, magazine, or the newspaper for a day. Use the time to meditate, walk in nature, work in the garden, nap, and watch a sunset. Whether you take half an hour or make it a day or weekend retreat, honor yourself with the gift of introspection. Reconnect your head to your body and pay attention to the sensations that correspond with your thoughts, and then trust them.

Practice introspection daily, for in the stillness is where we hear the gentle urgings of our heart and the profound guidance of our higher Self, God, or Great Spirit.

Padmasana (Lotus Pose) and Siddhasana (Perfect Pose)

Padmasana, also known as the Lotus Pose, is the classic seated posture for meditation; however, it must be approached with much practice and respect as it can be a very intense stretch in the knees. Siddhasana, also known as the Perfect Pose, is the preliminary asana that we practice to eventually achieve Padmasana. It does not require such a deep stretch in the knees but it does bring our bodies into a state of balance and prepares us for the Lotus. Both postures enhance concentration and are greatly revered as the best positions for pranayama and meditation.

> … Love plus meditation is compassion.
> —The Buddha

Energy is directed through the spine and around the body because of the crossed-leg connection which supports a straight and strong, yet supple spine. Turning our palms upward, either resting on our knees or in our lap, promotes the sense of accepting. Upturned hands with index finger and thumb touching keep the energy in our body clearly circulating, which causes us to concentrate at a deeper level.

These two postures are mostly what we think of when we visualize yoga or meditation, and rightly so. They both focus our concentration and turn our awareness inward to a more introspective and empowering observance.

As we practice the Perfect Pose or Lotus Pose, it is important to establish a grounded center from which to sit and then relax our body from the pelvic girdle while elongating our spine upward through the crown of the head while, at the same time, dropping into the base. As our body relaxes, our breath can flow more fully through our lungs. When this happens, we settle into an altered state of consciousness where nothing else matters but the present moment. This is true meditation.

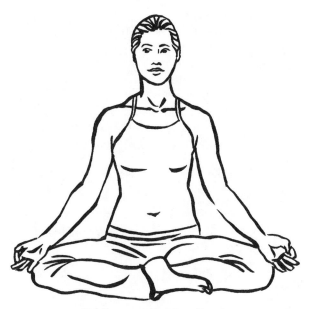

Siddhasana (Perfect Pose).

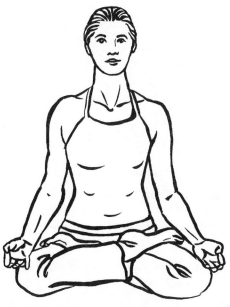

Padmasana (Lotus Pose).

Empowerment Exercise: Siddhasana/Padmasana

Siddhasana/Padmasana Affirmation: *Rooted in inner peace, I transcend to my higher Self.*

Although these two asanas are very similar, Siddhasana is a variation of Padmasana. It is recommended that you practice the Perfect Pose until you have enough experience and flexibility to attempt the Lotus Pose.

This first set of instructions describes Siddhasana:

1. Begin by sitting on the floor, legs extended and spread slightly apart.

2. Bend your left knee and slide your left heel into your groin area. Bend your right knee and place your right ankle directly over your left ankle and tuck your right foot between your left calf and hamstrings. Hook your left foot between your right calf and hamstrings.

3. Extend through your spine and sit tall, keeping your chin parallel to the floor.

4. Join your thumb and forefinger (jnana mudra) of each hand and extend the other three fingers directly out. Rest your hands, palms facing upward, on your knees.

5. Eyes may be open or closed as you breathe smoothly and naturally. You may also choose to incorporate Ujjayi Breath (see Chapter 7) while sitting in this posture.

6. To exit the pose, slide your top foot off the bottom leg and draw your knees up, rotating from the hips. Straighten both legs back in front of you.

Padmasana is considered the par excellence of the sitting poses:

1. Begin by sitting on the floor, legs extended. Bend your right knee, rotate the right hip outward, and cradle your right lower leg in the crooks of both elbows. Keep your torso straight and relax your hips. Place the right foot on top of your left thigh, close to your hip crease.

2. Lean back slightly and lift the left leg in front of the right. Carefully slide the left leg over the right leg, snuggling the edge of the left foot on top of the right thigh, close to the hip crease. Draw your knees as close together as possible, rotating from the hip joints.

3. Lift through the top of your sternum, relaxing into the hips, and place your hands in jnana mudra, thumb and forefinger touching, remaining fingers extended. Rest your hands on your knees, palms facing upward.

4. Breathe evenly. You may wish to use Ujjayi Breath. Never force yourself to stay in this posture longer than your body feels comfortable to do so. Start with three to five rounds of breath and work up from there as you are ready.

5. This is a two-sided pose, so repeat to the other side, beginning with your left leg this time.

Benefits

Both Siddhasana and Padmasana increase flexibility in the hips. They stimulate the pelvis, spine, abdomen, and bladder, although Padmasana's effects are somewhat deeper than Siddhasana. The first three chakras are stimulated in these two postures; however, all of the seven chakras are affected because of the increased energy moving through the spine.

These poses stretch the ankles and knees, which increases their flexibility to support the body while standing. Ankles especially tend to be forgotten when we do exercise of any kind, and Siddhasana/Padmasana bring our awareness to these most important areas.

Padmasana for women can be quite beneficial. It eases the discomfort caused by menstruation and also helps sciatic pain. Consistent practice of this pose until late into pregnancy is said to help ease the stress of childbirth.

Traditional texts say that Padmasana transforms all disease and awakens kundalini, the primordial energy of the Universe that lies dormant at the base of your spine.

Cautions

Considering the deep stretching through the knees and ankles in Siddhasana and Padmasana, it is wise to be mindful and only move your body as far as it wants to go. You may even decide that the Lotus Pose is not for you at this time. If so, don't worry that you can't do it now. Just continue to practice the Perfect Pose until one day your body will let you know that you are ready for Padmasana.

When entering these poses, be mindful not to twist or rotate your knees. Let all the rotation come from your hip joints. Padmasana is considered to be an intermediate to advanced posture, so it is wise to be respectful of this pose's intensity. Do not perform this pose without sufficient prior experience. You may also want to have the supervision of a trusted yoga teacher.

Real Life

Here are a few thoughts from one of my university students. With many years of experience in the study of meditation and yoga, Jim comes to class on his lunch hour with a great attitude and a willingness to see where his practice takes him.

"I have always had a competitive streak that at times serves a good purpose but in many situations is counterproductive for me. The noncompetitive nature of yoga really is a great blessing in regard to this attitude. Yoga has taught me that often the path to accomplishment is being in the moment and concentrating on what is happening instead of striving toward a goal. The goals will come through practice and patience. Many things in life can't be rushed and yoga teaches me this lesson very well.

What is meant to be will be. It isn't meant to be, I can't force it. No posture teaches me this more than Padmasana (Lotus).

I would love to sit in Padmasana to meditate. However, I am one of those people whose knees are nearly a foot off the floor in Baddha Konasana, so patience and practice are the key words if I'm ever going to be able to sit comfortably in Lotus. I try to remember to surrender, to try but don't strive and let my muscles, ligaments, and tendons stretch. That is when my body will change. If I attempt to force the changes, I will only end up injuring myself and putting the goals even farther from my grasp. I still have many lessons to learn on the mat.

Yoga has put me back in touch with parts of myself that have been buried for years. I am more comfortable, less stressed, and I find that my day-to-day life is better, easier. I remember the value of not being critical of everything either others or I do. I let people be who they are. I strive for good deeds and positive results but I don't get frustrated when things don't work out or if everyone doesn't share my views. Ram Dass said it best in his book *Be Here Now*."

Empowerment Journal

Stephen gives a wonderful example of how he has become more aware of his internal dialogue and how he has changed some of his negative thoughts and feelings about himself into more loving ways of being. Because of yoga, he has started truly listening to his inner thoughts and has begun to transform his life through the practice of stillness:

Yoga has empowered me in several ways. It has made me physically more healthy and active. I didn't exercise regularly before doing yoga, but now I walk, cycle, and take regular yoga classes as part of my life. I have more confidence in my physical capabilities now.

I have become more aware of my body and how good it can feel. My yoga practice has strengthened and straightened it out so that it is comfortable and I even feel more attractive in my body. I did not hate my body before, but I did not like it either, and liking it means I can see it as an integral part of myself rather than as a device that houses my spirit.

This integration of body and spirit has led to a meditation practice that I did not have before I started doing yoga. I now understand more deeply the body/mind/spirit union that meditation brings to me. One extraordinary fact that I have found is that I am more comfortable with silence and can find a place of "being" rather than "doing" all the time. This makes it easier for me to handle stress. It's easier for me to identify when I am stressed and use the breathing techniques and postures to help combat my discomfort. It is certainly a growth to be able to recognize when I am stressed and what is causing it. I am much more aware of my stress and now I have a way to relieve it.

My yoga practice is just beginning to teach me about living in the present moment, and it promises to help to relieve the stress of my "never-ending to-do list" outlook on life.

Mantras for Daily Living

Mantras and meditation go hand in hand. Many types of meditations already incorporate certain mantras such as Transcendental Meditation, known as TM or Primordial Sound Meditation taught by physician and author Deepak Chopra. These two types of meditations incorporate the use of Sanskrit syllables that are recited for the duration of the meditation to help keep the practitioner's mind from wandering. These particular mantras are specific to each individual and therefore have a very personal feeling to them.

Although it's not necessary to meditate with a mantra, they are excellent tools to help us focus. In particular, if there is something specific that you would like to instill in yourself like peace, concentration, or love, using a mantra as you meditate will enhance and support your intention.

I have listed some mantras that you may choose to create an inner state of peace and stillness. Take a few moments now, close your eyes, and breathe deeply as you recite one that resonates with you. If you already have your own special mantra, you are welcome to use it; however, don't be afraid to try something new. Read over the list, check in with your body and see which one resonates with you. You can even use a different mantra every time you meditate. Just remember the reason we use mantras is to instill a deeper awareness throughout our entire being. There are no wrong mantras but if you take the time to feel the right one for the moment, you will bring a deeper sense of clarity to your practice.

- "I am free from worry."
- "Relax, compassion, peace, love."
- "I am love."
- "Within me lies the power of stillness."
- "I am calm, I am still."
- "Om Mani Padme Hum." ("The jewel of consciousness is in the heart's lotus.")

This last mantra emphasizes that anything is possible when the heart and mind are connected. It is the most commonly recited mantra in the world.

Making the Time for Stillness

Now that we have the understanding and the tools for meditation, how do we find the time to actually practice? In our hectic and busy world there seems to be so much noise and activity around us that we find it hard to concentrate, much less find the time to just sit in stillness.

… get down from the head and into the heart and all problems disappear.
—Osho, existentialist and spiritual leader from India

There are many suggestions to assist us in creating stillness, but the main thing we must do is to commit to the time. We must allot ourselves a certain amount of time each day; whether it is 10 minutes or an hour, we must, without excuse, *y* the time. Once we have made that very important commitment to ourselves, then we can do many different things to enhance our experience of stillness.

If possible, create a space where you meditate. Come to this place on a daily basis. Use this space only for your meditations, if possible, because every act creates its own vibration, and by meditating in one place often, the space itself becomes meditative. Therefore, it will support you with each subsequent sitting and you will be able to go deeper into stillness each time you meditate.

Take the phone off the hook, put a "do not disturb" sign on the door, and treat your meditation space as sacred. Take your shoes off and leave them at the door. Leave all your preoccupations with your shoes and come to your sacred space with an open heart, an open mind, and a clear intention.

It's important to be comfortable, so don't force yourself to sit in a position that does not support you. You may even want to start meditating while walking if sitting is difficult for you. (If you choose a walking meditation, try to walk somewhere in nature without the pollution and noise of the city.) Most importantly, try not to have expectations about your practice. Simply let it be what it is.

Three essential components to meditation are relaxation, watching, and nonjudgment. As you incorporate these into your practice, a great stillness and peace will slowly descend over you. There is no wrong meditation as long as you show up for the practice, so be patient with yourself and be playful. Osho states "a really meditative person is playful." Allow yourself to feel the joy that comes with the understanding of who you really are.

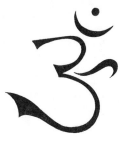

Chapter Eleven

Perfection in the Present Moment

Perfection is completeness beyond practical or theoretical improvement. It is entirely without any flaws, defects, or shortcomings. At this very second, there is perfection in this moment.

As esoteric as it sounds, when we can experience the present, completely aware of each moment, all of our troubles, fears, and doubts dissolve. In the present moment there is no past to feel guilty for, nor is there a future to worry about. There is only the now in which we exist.

Everything that we say or do is in the present moment. Think about it: We can't physically exist in the past or the future. All of our actions are performed in the now. We can remember the past or anticipate the future, but nothing gets accomplished in time that has already gone or that has not arrived. Through this understanding is how we find perfection in the present moment of just "being."

When we surrender our concerns of either the past or future and come to the present moment with an open heart and mind, we can begin to know peace. When our hearts and minds are filled with peace, we are open to experience the creativity and clarity of our soul.

Think of a time when everything seemed to fall into place and you felt that your life was perfect. I can remember my first trip to Hawaii. It was an unexpected vacation and very spontaneous, which helped me not worry about the future. It was magic. I allowed myself to be drawn into the adventure, experiencing with all five of my senses. With each new heady aroma and beautiful sight, I believed my life was perfect! There were no worries about how I was going to afford the trip and I didn't think about the problems that already existed. In short, I experienced each present moment as it arrived and fully lived the perfection in each second.

Yoga is perfection in the present moment. As we fold into a forward bend or extend through a Camel Pose, our full attention is in the presence of the posture. We support the movement with our breath and experience the physical and emotional releases through focusing on each present moment. There is a simple yet profound liberation in releasing all attachments from the past and future and surrendering into the present. In our surrender we find perfection.

Samadhi

Samadhi is the last limb of Patanjali's Yoga Sutras and has been referred to as a state of ecstasy. The previous two sutras, dharana (concentration) and dhyana (meditation) are essential to help us reach this state of pure bliss, because a one-pointed focus in meditation allows us to release from the limitations of the mind and body enough to reach a glimpse of enlightenment.

> Samadhi is perfect union of the individualized soul with the Infinite Spirit.
> —Paramahansa Yogananda, author of *Autobiography of a Yogi*

Sages throughout time have been practicing yoga, pranayama, and meditation to reach samadhi. Liberation from our mind and physical body is not easily attained, especially in this day and age of high technology, more work, and less free time. However, during those moments that we glimpse the freedom of our spirit we understand how ecstatic and pure is the feeling.

In samadhi, our crown chakra is opened to the enlightenment of oneness. We can feel our connection to God, to our higher Self, to Spirit.

Our ego dissolves and we understand that we are one with all life. This encompasses all beings and goes beyond time, space, and our three-dimensional reality. Samadhi is a state of grace and is the purest awareness known to human consciousness. At this level there is no separation between self and the "Self" because all is seen as one.

We are prone to think of samadhi as a purely mental state, which is not the case. This altered mystical state of consciousness can have a significant effect on our nervous system and the rest of the physical body as well as our mental state. As we release into relaxation at the end of our asana routine through Savasana, the Corpse Pose, all the systems of the body relax into homeostasis, releasing resistance and tension. This is a time for deep healing as well as the opportunity for enlightenment.

It's important to realize that the release of ordinary consciousness does not mean unconsciousness. On the contrary, while in samadhi, we are keenly aware, but without the distractions of attachment. We don't identify ourselves with anything, but we accept that we are completely one with everything. When we achieve a state of enlightenment, we know our spirit is eternal and is always at peace.

Integration

I use the word "integration" quite often while teaching classes to explain what happens when our breath coincides with our body. Integration is the act of combining into a unified and harmonious whole. Its meaning naturally supports the concept and practice of yoga. Through the integration of our yoga practice, we combine our breath and movement to create the physically, mentally, and emotionally beneficial effects of the asanas. Continuing with your yoga practice, you may become aware of physical changes taking place in your body. As you do, can you feel how these adjustments to your body affect your emotions, making you more conscious of the mind/body connection?

Once you awaken to the reality that you are responsible for your own life, you come to realize that you are, in a larger sense, responsible for the entire human family.

—Dan Millman, author of *Way of the Peaceful Warrior*

As the body and mind are integrated through the breath, so are our past and future. Breath is the unifying force that makes our practice flow. It is considered that which brings us to the present moment by connecting our past and future and also is the ingredient of our life, which connects our internal awareness to the outside world.

Our yoga practice is constantly asking us to become more aware of ourselves—not just our bodies but also our mind, emotions, and our very nature. The real value of asana practice is much more than a physically toned body or a spiritually clear mind. The value is that it can teach us to turn inward and truly "feel" through integrating the body, mind, and spirit. As our sensitivity to our full being increases, life becomes more fulfilling because we can savor the uniqueness of each individual moment.

More importantly, through integrating body, mind, and spirit we also become more aware of what moves us toward our dharma and what takes us away from it. (Remember that dharma is our soul path, the reason we were born to earth in the first place.) Through integration we are empowered and more peaceful. We are more focused on our soul's path and are able to handle life's endless stream of challenges without feeling overwhelmed or fearful. As a result, we become more effective in all of our actions as well as in our stillness. Because of this sense of connection, our very presence begins to inspire and bring out the best in people around us. Remember, if you are wondering how you are doing in your yoga practice, look at your life and how you are living it more than how you are accomplishing particular postures.

The awareness we develop on the yoga mat affects everything from our internal balance to the way we treat our family and friends and how we approach our life. As we become more aware in our yoga practice, we move toward sensitivity, which changes our individual consciousness. Thus, our actions reflect our awareness. The changes in our own awareness influence the consciousness and the actions of everyone we meet. The work we do on ourselves is felt throughout the Universe, and slowly we shift the direction the world is taking.

On the surface this may sound a little grandiose. However, knowing that we are all connected, it is easy to see that when one soul makes a conscious effort, all are affected. We have the opportunity to become an advocate of peace as we integrate our mat practice with our daily life, thus becoming an advocate for harmony in the world.

When We Meet Face to Face

Sometimes looking in the mirror is not the easiest thing to do. We see the clear reflection of our self without pretense. There is nothing that can hide the reality of who we are.

Many of the faults you see in others are your own nature reflected in them. As the Prophet said, "The faithful are mirrors to one another."
—Rumi, poet

Sometimes our mirror isn't a piece of glass hanging on a wall. Most likely someone in our life is the mirror with which we clearly see our self. Is there someone in your life who seems to rub you the wrong way no matter what they do? They aren't necessarily a negative person but they just seem to get on your nerves. Ask yourself what it is about them that bothers you so much. Whenever I need a good dose of "humble pie," I do this little exercise for myself. Usually, after objectively observing why certain people get under my skin, I realize that I am irritated because those people exhibit the same traits that I do not like in myself. Whoa! That's a big realization. Upon closer look, my friend's lateness that drives me crazy is very similar to my own rushing around and tardiness. The ego I see in some of my colleagues is what I strive to release in me.

On the other hand, mirroring does not always entail showing us our negative traits. It also reveals to us all of the beautiful traits that we possess. Think of someone you truly admire and have an affinity toward, perhaps your spouse, a close friend, or even a notable public figure. What is it about them that you find attractive? What makes you feel connected with them? Do they always show kindness to others? Are they a diligent and honest worker? Maybe they just exhibit grace and style. Either way, take a look at yourself and see if you, too, have any of these traits you like in the people around you. It is very possible that you are seeing your own good qualities in the people you find attractive.

We are drawn to what we need to work on; therefore, it is inevitable that we seek out people and things in our life that make us think and question our ideas and values. At the same time, through mirroring we are reassured of our own good qualities and of the path we are following in life.

Let's take our yoga practice and see how it mirrors to us. More than any person or activity, yoga mirrors exactly to us who we are. It does not judge, nor does it exalt us. It merely shows us where we are at any given time in our life.

For example, when I first started yoga I was terrible at backward bending. Forward bends were easy for me and I felt very confident when the teacher called for those poses. However, when she called for a Standing Backward Bend or a Camel Pose I would silently groan and start chastising myself for not being able to accomplish them the way I wanted. When I finally realized that my body, through the yoga poses, was talking to me, I began to realize why I had difficulty with backward bends. As it turned out, not only were my back muscles weak and constricted, but my heart energy was low. I had been carrying around a lot of sadness and grief from some personal issues I had not acknowledged. Not only did yoga help to physically open my body to backward bending, but it released all that pent-up grief and sadness to reveal the issues I had hidden deep inside. It was a process of awakening and empowerment, but nonetheless, with each yoga class, it mirrored to me what I needed to look at in myself.

Give yourself a few minutes to contemplate who and what are mirroring to you in your life. The next time you practice yoga either in class or on your own, listen to your body as it moves through the asanas and ask yourself, "What is important for me to know about this posture?" Let the answers come to you through the sensations, feelings, and thoughts you have while in the pose. Take off the rose-colored glasses and look at yourself in the mirror, squarely in the eyes. Let the mirror of yoga bring you face to face with yourself.

Seeing God in Everything

What does God mean to you? There are many different definitions of the One Creative Energy or Life Force that animates all of existence. Some believe "He" is an all-powerful being that exists somewhere "up there" and outside and around our self. Others know God to be an all-knowing, all-powerful, loving energetic force that continually flows through all of creation. Whatever our belief, whether we see God as energy or as a man or even a woman, we are empowered by the thought that God is in everything.

The way of God is complex, He is hard for us to predict. He moves the pieces and they come somehow into a kind of order.

—Euripides, Greek playwright

It is important for each of us to know God in our own sense, to have a personal relationship with this being of unconditional love. Through our own relationship with God we will then know where He resides and how He animates our lives. Yoga is one of the most empowering ways to have a relationship with God. Through your practice you integrate your physical body with your mental and emotional bodies to awaken your Spirit. It is through this awakening that you can see God, the Universal Energy, in everything.

God is in the trees, the sky, a sunset, your lover's eyes, your child's voice. God is in the dried autumn leaves, a newborn kitten, a sudden inspiration, and even in the midst of sorrow. The presence of God is in your breath, among your thoughts, and expresses itself through your actions.

Our yoga practice is a powerful expression of God manifesting in each present moment. When our only focus is on our body, mind, and spirit connection, and not on the grocery list of chores we have to do, we can clearly see how we are animated with Life Force. During your next yoga class or practice, make the effort to stay present. Notice how you feel when you place your full attention on each asana that you attempt. Can you feel surrender, clarity, and most of all empowerment fill through your being? Can you feel the energy of a greater Source will you? See God in everything, including yourself.

Practice: Nature Hike

A good way for us to become empowered with and aware of our present moments and to find the connections that we have to all beings is to take a hike. Literally, take a hike or a walk in nature and become aware of all the life that surrounds you. You don't have to find some remote, backwoods place to take your walk. Utilize what is around you. If you live in the city, find a park and walk there. If you live near a body of water such as the ocean or a lake, walk around there. It doesn't really matter where you hike as long as you bring your attention to what is going on around you and how it is affecting you internally.

I have never been happier, more exhilarated, at peace, rested, inspired, and aware of the grandeur of the Universe and the greatness of God than when I find myself in a natural setting not much changed from the way He made it."
—Jimmy Carter, former president of the United States

For example, there is a wonderful small state park right in the heart of Nashville. I go there often to reflect, rejuvenate, and sometimes to be still. There are beautiful hiking trails, a wide variety of animal and bird life, many trees and flowers, and of course, fellow hikers.

As I make my way around the lake trail, I walk slowly so I can see the large spider webs hanging from the bamboo leaves, and hear the wood-peckers in the tree-tops and the owls hooting their calls at dusk. Many times I have shared moments with deer when we met face to face on the trails. I connect with the people I meet on these hikes, too. Whether I feel a positive energy from them or a negative one, I still feel energy coming from them, so this proves to me that we have some sort of energetic con-nection to each other.

Each time I connect with the hikers, animals, and even the plant life, I am empowered through a sense of unity. It feels as if there is an all-knowing consciousness between us. I choose to call this consciousness God. By taking the time for these nature hikes, I restore my own connection to my center, find stillness within, and thus create an open doorway to self-realization and empowerment.

Give yourself a gift and take a walk somewhere in nature. Open your eyes to all the life around you. Can you feel how alive and empowered you are just by absorbing this natural energy? Without judging it, watch it, hear it, sense it, and then recognize your connection with all creation.

Death Is Only a Condition

Are you surprised to see a section in a yoga book regarding death? Isn't our yoga practice supposed to be about enlightenment, empowerment, and "waking up" to our higher Self? Of course it is, and that is why death is such an integral part of our yoga practice and of living. It is a transition from one life to the next, from one way of perceiving our exis-tence to another, but mostly it is a surrender of our ego so it can merge with the higher consciousness of unconditional love. It is through this letting go of our own self-importance that we are able to reach our liberation, samadhi, and feel the connection we have with all of existence.

God's love is beyond death.
—Deepak Chopra, best-selling author and physician

So then, death of the ego is one of the things that yoga encourages us to achieve. We are releasing that part of us which keeps us separate from love, from freedom, and from unity. As we come to our yoga mat with loving respect for the movement of the asanas, ourselves, and all sentient beings, our ego begins to die, to transition into a selfless state. In this egoless state, when we move into any asana we are not our ego-self nor are we the body that is practicing. We are simply the understanding observer in the movement. There is no judgment of right or wrong and there is no pride of a job well-done.

This concept may sound a little strange considering that we do have a body with an ego and we are used to perceiving our world through that view. However, if we take a conscious step back to pratyahara (see Chapter 8) and dharana (see Chapter 9) to turn our awareness inward with a focused concentration, we can release the ego's mind control and come to stillness. Here we see the illusion of a separate self and let it disappear into the whole of existence. In that very moment, we die to the ego-self and transition to the consciousness of our higher Self.

If the thought of death is frightening to you, ask yourself why. What is the underlying cause for your fear? Are you afraid of nonexistence, or is it a fear of the unknown? These fears are rooted in the ego because it is trying to preserve an identity that is separate from the whole. Our ego serves a good purpose, but it tends to move past that purpose to create separateness and isolation in us when we don't look for and sense our connection to other beings. It can be released when we surrender ourselves to love, in our yoga practice and through humble service. The death of the ego fills us with more joy and empowerment than we can imagine.

Merging with Your Higher Self

Let's take our discussion regarding death to a deeper level and examine it as it applies to our yoga practice. We have already discussed that the ego must surrender its control over our lives in order for us to release the fear of death, but what about letting go on the yoga mat? If we come to our practice with the idea that we are going to "look better" than yesterday or outdo the guy next to us in class, then it will take some time for us to understand what yoga is all about. On the other hand, if we practice the asanas (postures) and pranayama (breath) with reverence and surrender, then our ego has no time to judge ourselves against our neighbor or our previous practice. Slowly, ego gives way to connection and trust. When we start to trust our own body we become more open to receiving guidance from it.

At first I did yoga, then yoga did me, now yoga *is* me.
—Anonymous

Once we can listen to our body and follow its inner promptings of movement, we can then deepen our connection between it and the mind and also our emotions. When you breathe deeply into the lowest part of your lungs, notice how the expansion of your torso connects with your mind. Is there anything specific you can think of when you feel fresh oxygen fill your lungs? An example might be that you think of energy and life when you breathe in but when you breathe out you contemplate letting go of stress.

How about your emotions, what happens to them when the body expands with a full breath? (Keep in mind that your mind can only interpret emotions, so try to stay in the "feeling" instead of the thought.) Do you feel free, peaceful, energetic, or even centered? Whatever your feeling, whatever your thoughts, know that through the movements of your body you are affecting your thoughts and feelings.

It is wise to be aware that this process works in all directions. Whatever we think and feel can have a major affect on our body, too. If our ego is constantly telling us that we can't do something and we feel that it is true, our body will have a difficult time in achieving the desired outcome.

The best way to empower our self and merge with our higher Self is to surrender. We must die to our ego and become completely trusting in our higher Self. As we trust our yoga practice to take us deeper into our body, so too can we trust that our practice will affect our whole life in a positive manner.

The poet Rumi so eloquently assures us that dying is in fact the beginning of life. He makes no excuses for the ego when he states, "Don't fear the death of that which is known. If you die to the temporal you will become timeless. Cut off those chains that hold you prisoner to the world of attachment. In the silence of love you will find the spark of life."

So let us come to our yoga practice with trust. Let go in loving detachment of our ego so that we may truly become empowered with the awareness that we are greater than our self because we are a part of the whole of creation, and in that whole everything is possible.

Savasana (Corpse Pose)

It is essential that our body is placed in a supine, neutral position in Savasana so that the energy can flow uninterrupted. This is our time to rejuvenate, to heal, and to realize our connection to our Divine Source, God. Savasana should conclude both our asana and pranayama practices as it helps to focus and integrate the work that we've done. As we rest in deep relaxation the cells of our body are "remembering" every posture that we moved through in our yoga practice. Every movement, every breath is being recorded into our cellular memory as we rest in Savasana. It is through this posture that we can reach that deep stillness, that complete awareness which gives rise to spiritual liberation, to the ecstasy that is samadhi.

Physically, Savasana slows our metabolism, decreasing our blood pressure and heart rate, which induces the relaxation response. It also calms our brain and helps to relieve stress, fatigue, and mild depression while strengthening the immune system. This pose gives us time to absorb and integrate all the postures of our previous practice. The physical responses of this asana help to integrate the mental and emotional effects as well, thus enabling us to experience that deeply relaxed state that releases our identification with the body/mind so we can experience a clear connection with our soul.

Even though this pose is one of relaxation and stillness, it is said to be the most difficult posture to attain. While the body is completely relaxed, the mind is free from chatter and our awareness is keen. It is difficult for many of us to attain this focused yet completely surrendered state. Either we have relaxed into unconsciousness so deeply that we fall asleep or our mind is unable to slow down enough to release tension from the body. However, it is important not to judge ourselves if we do not immediately reach samadhi while in Savasana. Every time we come to Savasana we achieve the benefits of rejuvenation, and with practice we will find that we are able to move closer to ecstasy with our Savasana practice.

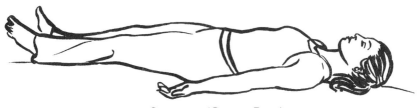

Savasana (Corpse Pose).

Empowerment Exercise: Savasana

Savasana Affirmation: *I surrender to the awareness and power of the present moment.*

Savasana can be a most transformational experience; however, to the beginning yoga student it can prove to be a bit of a challenge. Through the Corpse Pose we attempt to bring our mind and body into stillness through deep relaxation. At the same time, we rest in conscious awareness that encompasses the present moment. For many of us, that centered, conscious stillness is elusive. Perhaps we have occasionally slipped into that pure awareness and when we have, the experience was profound and memorable. In those moments, we have glimpsed spiritual liberation and surrendered to the ecstasy of samadhi.

1. Lie on your back with knees bent. Tuck your tailbone in and relax your lower back into the floor. Then, one by one, lower your legs to the floor away to lengthen your spine. Let your feet rest about hip width apart, allowing your toes to relax to the side.

2. Stretch your shoulders down and away from your ears. Move your shoulder blades down your back, but keep them spread apart on the floor. Turn the palms of your hands upward to open the shoulders. Rest your arms at your sides.

3. Tuck your chin toward your Adam's apple, then soften your neck and facial muscles.

4. Close your eyes and gaze toward your third eye (the point between your eyes). Begin to notice the rhythm of your breath.

5. Begin Ujjayi Breath (see Chapter 7), following the path of your breath inward and outward until you no longer focus on your breath but on pure awareness itself.

6. To return to an upright position, slowly wiggle your toes, fingers, hands, and feet to orient yourself back to your present circumstances. Draw your knees to your chest and roll onto your right side. Push up from the right side and come to a comfortable cross-legged position.

Benefits

Savasana is the king of relaxation poses. It activates the "relaxation response" by slowing down the body's metabolism. This helps to reduce chronic high blood pressure when practiced two times per day for at least ten minutes.

This pose should be included in every asana practice. We should try to begin and end our yoga workout with this pose as it brings our bodies to a centered, focused state where we move with intention and awareness. When practiced at the end of a yoga class, this pose integrates the effects of our entire practice, thus helping our bodies to rejuvenate and heal themselves.

Physically, our bodies let go into deeper states of relaxation. Pain seems to ease or disappear during our Savasana practice. Some practitioners have even stated that they no longer felt their bodies while they were in this state of deep relaxation. Others explained they feel a sense of floating.

On the mental level, the needless chatterings and negative self-talk disappear, or at least they fade into the backs of our minds. When we can enter a state of "nothingness" and rest there, we have achieved the pure effects of Savasana.

Emotionally, we are able to surrender to whatever feeling we are experiencing. This is not to say that we hide from or stuff our emotions back inside, but we allow them to float up to the surface without fear or attachment to them. This can be quite liberating when we rest in a state of "being" in the present moment and do not concern ourselves with ego.

The benefits of Savasana are many and profound. Give yourself the gift of experiencing this pose beyond all poses.

Cautions

One of the best parts of this posture is there are no real cautions. This pose is considered the most difficult to master, yet it is such a relaxing and opening posture. Perhaps the difficulty rests more with the mind than the body. This asana was meant to release the chatter of the mind and to bring it to stillness so that we can reach enlightenment through samadhi. Many of us have some difficulty stopping our thoughts when we try to relax, and find this pose to be somewhat of a struggle.

On a physical note, it is not advised that pregnant women lie in Savasana after their first trimester as the weight of the baby puts pressure on the nerves of the spine. This can cause discomfort and may cause other problems. Please check with your doctor if you have questions regarding this.

If you are pregnant, finish your practice resting in side-lying Savasana with cushions under your head and between your knees. It is not advised, however if you still prefer resting on your back try doing so for very short periods of time.

Real Life

A longtime student of mine and yoga enthusiast, Patrick, shares his story of an experience he had while in Savasana. He was able to experience the sensation of pure consciousness, feeling himself connected with everything; as with most of us, he was able to rest in this awareness for a few minutes. The wonderful proof that yoga is integrated throughout Patrick's life is that he has the ability to draw upon his experiences from class—in particular Savasana—and apply them to his daily life when he needs it the most. Read on for a glimpse into complete consciousness.

"For me, the highlight of each yoga class is Savasana at the end of the evening. Through this posture, I have developed an appreciation and understanding of the power of a single breath and I have become more and more attuned to my body/mind connection.

Savasana is more than a deep relaxation. My creative visualizations transport me to a dreamlike state, almost as if I were slumbering. However, I am completely aware of my body and my surroundings while I am resting in Savasana.

The most striking Savasana experience I have had was at the end of the deep relaxation when the sound of the chimes resonated through the room and passed through me like ripples on a pond. I felt as if I was as fluid as water. I carried that sensation with me for the rest of that evening.

Now, in my day-to-day life, I can take a deep breath, physically and mentally re-center myself, and recapture a moment of my experiences in Savasana."

Empowerment Journal

It's time to check in with your empowerment journal. How is it coming along? Remember not to judge yourself with this tool, but to use it to make you more aware of your personal progress. Think of it as your mirror. The experiences you share in your journal ultimately give you clues to the progress you are making in your life.

To love oneself is the beginning of a life-long romance.
—Oscar Wilde, English poet, playwright, and novelist

Kathi is a certified Ashtanga Yoga instructor and has been practicing for quite some time. Her devotion to yoga and the practice of self-awareness is a sweet thing to witness. I feel fortunate to know her and to share her thoughts and experiences regarding Savasana:

Savasana has been referred to as the "Heart of Yoga." I agree whole "heartedly." I connected to my heart during Savasana the very first time I entered it.

I used to be one of those people who fell into the trap of self-judgment, self-criticism, self-hatred, and all-around self-abuse because I never thought I could measure up to the high standards I set for myself. Somehow during my life I became too busy to become still, and it was literally killing me.

It was during my first Ashtanga Yoga class that I was able to release my self-inflicted dis-ease and begin to accept myself, in body, mind, and spirit, for who I am.

During Savasana is when I make a conscious connection with God. It is during my yoga practice that I surrender, observe, and absorb the endless physical benefits and consequently, emotional peace. In Savasana, my physical body melts, my mind becomes still, and it is then that I become one with God. I come to a place where there is no right or wrong, no judgment or criticism, just pure and total love.

Mantras for Daily Living

Practices such as fasting, silence, vision quests, yoga, meditation, and prayer have all been used throughout time to deepen our connection to God, our Divine Source. The purpose of these disciplines is to keep us grounded in our body and clear in spirit. Mantras, especially, increase our focus in these practices and can deepen the experience.

As we focus on our crown chakra in this chapter, I have offered mantras that relate to our connection with our Divine Source as well as to all beings. Read through this list, taking your time to feel your responses with these mantras and find if any resonate with you. Feel free to alter this list or use your own mantras to stimulate your seventh energy center, which is the connection to God, our Divine Self.

Even if your life doesn't feel the way you would like it to be right now, ask yourself "What's good about this?" and watch your mind go to work, looking for something good in your life. Tell yourself that you are happy to be experiencing your daily routine and then reinforce your gratefulness with a mantra that supports you in your daily life as well as in your spiritual awareness.

- "I honor and respect my divine Spirit."
- "God is in me, above me, below me, and around me at all times."
- "I am connected to *all* beings."
- "I am love, I am light, I am Spirit."
- "My soul rests in conscious awareness."
- "I am 'one' with all that is."
- "I give thanks for ... (your personal gratitude)."

Namasté: We Are All *"One"*

Every culture has a way in which they greet one another. In many places it is customary to shake hands or bow in greeting. In many places in the Far East, however, the customary greeting is full of honor and respect and the acknowledgment behind the gesture can have a deep spiritual connotation. Many Western yoga practitioners have also adopted this greeting and incorporate it into their practice as well as their entire life.

We place our hands together in the prayer position and gently press them toward our chest as we bow our head and say "Namasté": "I honor you as I honor myself. I acknowledge we are all *One*." This gesture is an acknowledgement of our connection to the other person and is a statement of honor and respect to them. In performing this greeting, we are recognizing the sacred space of another person and realizing our own space, knowing that everyone is equal, whole and beautiful in the eyes of the Universe.

I close every class that I teach with "Namasté" and the accompanying meaning to honor my students as well as myself for taking the time to practice and to share with the whole group. It is a loving and nurturing way to close our time together and to bring the class to full circle. For me personally, it is a constant reminder that although we all have different qualities and abilities, we are in fact, brothers and sisters of the Universe, connected in spirit. When I can see another person in that manner, then I can see the beauty within and honor them. This also helps me to be less judgmental and more accepting of another person's viewpoints and idiosyncrasies. In turn, I can be more loving and accepting of myself, too, which empowers me and allows me to be centered in the present. When I can see all of creation as equal then I have no more need to control or resist the outcomes of life.

Can you think of someone you have been having problems understanding and accepting because they look at life much differently than you? Maybe neither one of you can see eye to eye and are having problems even being kind to each other. The next time you start to feel the frustration of your differences, try bringing your hands together in the prayer position (anjali mudra) and state "I honor you as I honor myself. I acknowledge we are one," or simply say "Namasté." Either say it directly to them if you feel comfortable and safe doing so, or say it to yourself, directing the intention toward them.

Notice how you feel after you place your intention. Do you feel lighter, more empowered, less agitated, and more at peace? Continue practicing this gesture and notice how you become more accepting of your life and the people in it. Also recognize how this small gesture, this yoga mudra (hand position) changes you internally. With practice and dedication, you will come to feel a sense of internal peace and empowerment because of the unconditional love that is growing inside of you.

Yoga does not always have to be grand gestures and asanas that tone our bodies. Some of its greatest benefits come to us through integration of body, mind, and spirit and surrendering into stillness so that we may feel our connection to God, Great Spirit, and realize that we are all *One*.

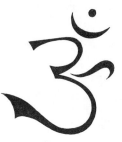

Chapter Twelve

Being a Fully Alive Person

What does being fully alive actually mean? Most people would agree that you're either alive or you're not. In one sense, this statement is true; however, in the realization of our full potential, it falls far short. It's possible that we can be alive, breathing (barely), walking through life, doing what we have to do without knowing joy and the excitement of discovery. Wouldn't you rather enjoy adventure, surprises, recognition, and even contentment and peace?

Many people don't realize that is exactly what life is all about! When I was living in Phoenix, I had a friend who was 10 years old. His father, grandparents, and sister were sitting around the living room contemplating what they had to do for the day. When Jay bounded into the room, his grandfather asked him what he was going to do that day. His reply was the wisest and most honest answer anyone could ever give. Jay said to his grandpa, "I'm gonna play, play, play!"

That's it! We have to play in life, not work ourselves silly until we can't enjoy our own existence! It's true that we have responsibilities to our family, our job, our community, and even our country, but our most important responsibility is to our self and our spiritual, emotional, mental, and physical health. When we are unable to access love for our self then we have nothing to give others. We are merely existing in our life without fully living it.

Don't let self-sacrifice confuse you. If you deny yourself something because you truly wish to give love to another being, then you have denied yourself nothing because love is expansive and affects the giver as well as the recipient. However, if you deny yourself for another's comfort and you feel used, left out, and even thankless, then you did not give love. Judgment, force, and expectation were given instead, and you will feel them returning to you as well.

It's time to be fully alive! Experience your life as a playground in which you experience everything from the swings to the merry-go-round to the monkey bars where you can hang upside down and see life from a different angle. In the words of my sweet friend Jay, "play, play, play!"

Beginner's Mind

We all know what it's like to begin something new. There is a sense of excitement, adventure, anticipation, and even uncertainty that takes over our senses. It seems there is something new to learn every time we turn around. When we are learning new things and applying them to our lives, we have focus and a conscious desire to educate our self further. Beginner's mind is pure and open and does not have any expectations or judgments.

I had no idea what to expect when I walked into my very first yoga class. The only thing I knew was I needed this class to graduate from college and I did have a sense of adventure for trying something that was out of the ordinary for my life. As I waited for the instructor to begin, I remember thinking that I was about to learn something new and I felt some anticipation but had no idea what I was getting myself into. Looking back on that feeling now, it makes me smile to think how exciting it was then to try something new.

The idea of beginner's mind in yoga—and in all of life—is to never let it go from your consciousness. Approach everything in your life with the enthusiasm, dedication, and focus of a beginner. You may be wondering how you can think like a beginner in your yoga practice when you've been taking classes for years. After all, you know all the names of the postures and you know how to move through them. Beginner's mind has nothing to do with relearning what you know but everything to do with having the excitement and dedication in your practice now that you had when you first started.

Think of the first yoga class you ever took. Do you remember the sense of adventure you felt as you walked into the room for the first time, set up your mat, and waited to begin class? What thoughts were going through your mind? Were you nervous, excited, peaceful, open to all possibilities? Because you didn't have anything to compare it to, you had no idea of what to expect. Instead, you participated fully, eager to see what was coming next. Each posture was a new experience for your physical body as well as for your mind and your emotions.

As with your yoga practice, you can apply beginner's mind to every aspect of your life. Empower yourself in the workplace with enthusiasm and anticipation. Even if you've been doing your job for years, find a new angle of seeing the fun in the work you do.

Rejuvenate and excite your relationships with your children, your spouse, your friends, and even yourself as you rediscover their unique qualities that bring you joy, love, and fulfillment. Let each day bring something new for you to discover with each of your relationships. Take the staleness out of your daily routine by changing the way you look at it. As you change your perceptions and drop your expectations, you will experience beginner's mind more often, which will empower your life with enthusiasm, creativity, and more love for yourself and the people in your life.

This mind-set is not rigid, so allow yourself to change directions and change your mind when you need to. Look at life as if everything is always new regardless of how many times you've experienced it before. See life through the eyes of a child. Get up early to watch a sunrise. Love yourself for being a novice at certain things. Don't try to do everything right on the first try. Jump up and down and get excited when you do!

Forgive yourself. Allow yourself to start over whether it is a major life lesson or a small task. Have compassion and patience with yourself and others. Above all, remember that you can have "beginner's mind" with your second chances, so be loving to yourself and know that every chance is an opportunity to see life anew.

Rediscovering Joy on a Daily Basis

Joy fills our life when we are connected to others. This connection has no limits, nor strict definitions. Every relationship that we have—whether it is with our lover or spouse, parents, children, friends, colleagues, acquaintances, and even animals and inanimate objects—is an opportunity for joy. Most importantly, the relationship we have with our self is the key factor in experiencing joy throughout our life.

Let yourself be silently drawn by the stronger pull of what you really love.
—Rumi, poet

How we experience our world all comes back to how we perceive it. If we look at our life and see it as struggle and pain, loss, and judgment, it will be very difficult to find any joy to sustain us. However, if we see our world as a collection of large and small miracles and take responsibility for own actions, we will view our world with love, respect, and abundance, and most significantly, we will experience empowerment, deep happiness, and peace in the acceptance of what "is." This is true joy.

Think of a time when someone you love did something unexpectedly nice for you. Maybe she presented you with a gift for no special reason except for the fact that she loved you. Perhaps a friend just called to say he was thinking of you and wanted you to know he cares. Maybe your husband, without warning, turned to you and said you were the most beautiful woman in the world, or your wife slipped a note in your briefcase to say that she loves you. How did it feel to receive love from someone else? Did you experience happiness, surprise, comfort, and most of all joy?

Remember a time when you performed acts of kindness for others. You might have sent a donation to the rescue mission or even volunteered some of your time to help out, or maybe you brought your special homemade chocolate chip cookies to the office to share with your colleagues. Think about all the times you prepared your children's lunches for school, and how you included special treats to surprise them when they opened their lunchboxes. Remember the times you surprised your spouse with indications of your love like notes on the pillow, a phone call in the middle of the day to say "I love you," a special dinner prepared and ready for when he or she walked through the door after work. Notice how every one of those acts of love made you feel. There was joy in your giving.

Joy permeates giving and receiving because of the love behind it. When we can be conscious of and openly give and receive loving-kindness throughout our lives, we then rediscover joy and the fullness of a peaceful, happy, and empowered life.

You Are Everything You Need

One of the aspects of being a fully alive person is trusting that everything we need is within our self. Of course, we rely on our interactions with others to make our life easier, but there is nothing that we need outside of our self to make us an empowered person. As we wake up to our true nature, our higher Self, we come to realize that because we are connected to all of creation, the source of our sustenance is endless.

Everything in the Universe is within you. Ask all from yourself.
—Rumi, poet

Many of us make the mistake of feeling that we will be truly happy when we marry a certain person or have a child by a certain age or achieve a specific career goal. We may think empowerment has to do with control and financial wealth. On the contrary, none of these things will bring empowerment and happiness (although it is possible that they can enhance what we already have). If we are content with our life and feel good about who we are, then marrying the right person or having a child can be wonderfully joyful and empowering experience. However, if we feel empty and lonely and desperate to find security, a spouse or a child cannot change how we feel inside. In fact, it is quite possible that they could exaggerate your feelings of desperation.

The key to empowerment and happiness is to find it within your self. To do that you must get to know your self better. Don't be afraid to ask your self questions and look for the answers if you don't already know them. There is nothing wrong with not knowing what you want out of life if you are willing to find out what you desire and then go for it! The more you know your self, the better able you will be to choose wisely the people, experiences, and perceptions of your life.

Ask Yourself Questions

It is good to ask questions. This is how we gain insight into others and our own thought processes. Asking our self questions can be an empowering experience from the standpoint of knowing our self more deeply. Our questions don't have to always be drawn-out philosophical ponderings, although they can give us immense food for thought.

Go to your bosom; Knock there, and ask your heart what it doth know.
—William Shakespeare, English playwright and poet

A good example of asking yourself a simple question is to just ask yourself how deeply you are breathing in the present moment. By bringing your awareness to your breath, you consciously realize how your body is reacting to the situations you find yourself in. If your breath is shallow, ask yourself why and then take a deep breath and become aware of your surroundings.

Our yoga practice is a wonderful place to ask simple questions to achieve deep results. As you move into each asana, continually ask yourself how you're feeling. Are your muscles stretching easily? Is your breath full and even? Can you take your stretch a little deeper? Don't forget to ask your heart and emotions what is going on. Are you feeling a little anxious in a standing backward bend, or can you feel a release of tension in your heart? Does forward bending make you feel safe? What emotions come up for you in certain postures?

You can see that all of these questions lead to deeper insights to help you understand yourself better. Through this clearer understanding of our self we come to know what we want out of life and how we hope to achieve it. As we know our self better, we can understand the people in our life more and therefore create and sustain more empowered and loving relationships.

Our body is the best place to start when asking our self questions. It will never lie, and it gives tangible insights. Ask yourself questions and then be open to hear the answers and apply them to your life.

Practice: Forgiveness

A practical aspect of understanding our self better and becoming a fully alive person is the practice of forgiveness. You may be wondering what forgiveness has to do with being fully alive, but it may surprise you at how empowered you feel once you forgive yourself and others for whatever it is that has offended you.

> He who knows others is learned; He who knows himself is wise.
> —Lao Tzu, Chinese philosopher and founder of Taoism

In our journey through life we have constant opportunities to choose forgiveness and to release negative thoughts and feelings about others and our self. As we let go of the mental negativity we may be holding, we in turn release the physical repercussions of our thoughts and emotions and are able to be comfortable in the present moment. When we forgive we let go of the guilt and slights of the past, which enables us to experience a sense of freedom and empowerment in the present.

This ceremony can help us take a step toward forgiving others and our self and thus enable us to become alive and fully actualized. On a piece of paper, list the grievances you hold against others and the things you need to forgive in yourself. Hold this list in your hands and ask your higher self to help you release all of the grudges, anger, hurt feelings, and pain to the highest good of all involved. Then burn the piece of paper or tear it into tiny pieces, saying out loud "I forgive and I am forgiven." A small symbolic act opens the door for internal transformation, and by creating a ceremony, you confirm your commitment to choosing forgiveness, but most of all you affirm your right to live life to the fullest and greatest potential of your being.

Looking at Life from a Different View

Perceptions are the most important consideration as to the way we see life. As a matter of fact, no two people will experience life in the same way. Our experiences have nothing to do with what actually happens to us but everything to do with how we perceive them.

The only true need anyone has is to be seen as real.
—Deepak Chopra, best-selling author and physician

For example, let's say two women go to the same yoga class. They both are about the same age and have a similar build. However, one woman has never practiced yoga before and has a history of tight hips and hamstrings. The other woman in class has been a yoga practitioner for many years and is in very good physical shape. How do you think these two women will experience the class?

The woman who has never taken a yoga class before may have the experience of beginner's mind. She may perceive yoga as a refreshing and exciting class, noticing many new and different sensations throughout her body. Since her hips and hamstrings were tight to begin with, she may think that yoga is a strenuous workout and wonder if she can keep up with the class. She may even be surprised at the emotions that express themselves in her. It is quite possible that she would have many thoughts running through her mind as she processes her new experiences. Thus, her perception of yoga might be that it is difficult yet refreshing.

The second woman, on the other hand, may have a completely different experience. Since she has been practicing for a longer period of time and her body reflects the workouts, she may come to class with less excitement but more contentment. Her body already has a sense of how yoga feels and she therefore trusts the experience more than the first woman might. The second woman's perceptions of yoga may be more nurturing and she may have a greater understanding of the process because she has a longer history with it.

Both women's perceptions are correct for their experiences. One is not better than the other, however; they are just different. If we can be open to other people's ideas and viewpoints, their perceptions of life, then we can broaden our own experiences of living. It is a wise and empowered person who allows others to have their own perceptions but who does not believe those perceptions to be his or her own.

When Life Turns Upside Down

When life turns upside down and brings us unwanted challenges, as it often does, we may try to force certain things to happen or coerce people to do what we want. These actions arise from fear and insecurity and they shut us off from our feelings. The opposite of feeling is force. When we force situations, we cannot feel from our heart. In essence, we have closed ourselves off from the connection we share with all beings and, in turn, we begin to force our will and lose awareness of the effect our efforts have on our own personal life and on other people involved. By forcing our will, we lose inner power and become internally weak, unable to find strength in ourselves. Forcing makes us angry and inflexible, and raises our blood pressure.

Life, I fancy, would very often be insupportable, but for the luxury of self-compassion.

—George Gissing, English novelist and critic

Releasing into our feelings, on the other hand, makes us calmer, more receptive, and more understanding of our situations and the people involved. In turn, this helps to make us physically, emotionally, and mentally healthier. People who have the security that comes with deep sensitivity and awareness have no desire to be violent. Insecurity contributes to violence and violence is merely a secondary characteristic of fear.

When I experience times of anger, fear, and insecurity, I turn to pranayama and yoga. Filling my lungs with deep yogic breaths helps to calm my mind and lower my blood pressure, which in turn eases my anger and fear. As I move through my yoga practice and focus only on the present moment, I feel the negative emotions leave my body and mind. I have found yoga to be one of the best ways to release fear, and thus re-establish trust in myself and my surroundings.

The next time you feel yourself beginning to get angry, take a few deep breaths and exhale them slowly. Ask yourself what is the cause of your anger or fear. Once you can identify the source of your stress, you can let it go and return to that peaceful, calm place within. From there you can feel your life turn right side up once again.

Sirsasana (Headstand Pose)

Sirsasana is known as the king of the asanas. Many yoga students aspire to this posture thinking it is very difficult and nearly impossible to achieve without years of practice. However, as your balance improves, this pose becomes very easy to accomplish. You will be surprised how easy it is to stand in this asana once you find the mental and physical balance to bring to the pose.

It's true this is not a pose for beginning students, but it should not be looked upon as something you could not accomplish with practice.

I was five years old when I attempted my first yoga headstand. It definitely was not the most graceful or precise pose I have ever done, but it was a start! Every day after kindergarten I would come home and turn the television on, excited to watch *Sesame Street* (it was a brand-new kid show at the time!). Lilias Folan had a slot on PBS that aired just before *Sesame Street* so I would catch the last part of her show, too. At first, being a five year old I had no idea what she was doing, but it looked fun because she would put her body in all sorts of funny positions! I didn't really pay attention to what she was saying, but I began to follow her actions until one day I found myself doing a headstand with her. At first I kept falling over backwards, over and over, until I finally tried again and this time held the pose for probably three seconds until I fell over backwards again. That was enough for me, though, and from then on I was hooked! It was kind of fun to flip over and think of myself as walking on the ceiling instead of the floor.

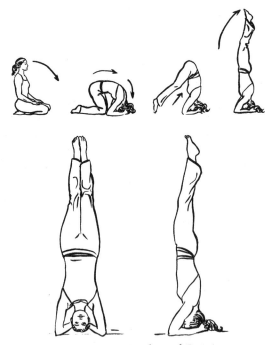

Sirsasana (Headstand Pose).

If we can bring our inner child to our practice, our free as a bird, excited to be alive little one with us to our yoga mat, it will encourage us to be more adventurous and take more risks for the fun of it.

So approach Sirsasana with adventure and respect. Trust in the abilities of your body and let go of your ego and mental chatterings and try looking at your world with a different view.

Empowerment Exercise: Sirsasana

Sirsasana Affirmation: *I live my life with a light heart and open mind.*

It's important to note that you may do this posture next to a wall for support. Repeat the entire instructions while facing a wall. Be sure to give yourself enough space away from the wall for you to lift your legs comfortably.

1. Begin by sitting in Vajrasana, knees bent, sitting on your heels. Bend forward, placing your forearms on the floor in front of you. Clasp your fingers together, making a triangle between your elbows and hands. Your elbows are shoulder width apart.

2. Place the top of your head on the floor between your hands.

3. Tuck your toes under and straighten your legs as if coming into the Dolphin Pose. Walk your feet toward your head, keeping the weight in your forearms. There should be only a very small amount of weight on your head.

4. Extend through your neck and shoulders, moving the blades down your back. Press into your arms and feel the weight shift into your upper body.

5. Tuck in your stomach (this pose is contingent in large part on the stomach), lifting your knees toward your chest. You may lift one leg at a time to begin with, eventually lifting both legs together. Move slowly, checking in with your head, neck, shoulders, and spine.

6. Bring your feet overhead as you press your forearms into the floor. Continue tucking your stomach, supporting your lower back. Be mindful not to tip your tailbone out, which can arch the back. Tuck your tailbone under to support your lower back.

7. Breathe deeply, and soften your gaze and facial muscles. Maintain this posture as long as you feel comfortable doing so.

8. To release from the pose, lower your legs slowly, come back to your knees, and rest in Child's Pose to counter the Headstand.

Benefits

Sirsasana develops an inner sense of balance and strength. It reverses any negative effects of gravity in that the heart is lower than the rest of the body and does not have to work as hard to pump blood throughout the body. This increases blood supply to the upper body, especially the brain. Because it is easier for blood to flow toward the upper body in this asana, Sirsasana stimulates the brain and helps to relieve fogginess and develops poise and lightness. It also improves memory and concentration.

This posture has even been known to relieve varicose veins by releasing gravity and relieving the pressure in the legs.

If ever you are upset or disillusioned with your life, turn upside down and look at the world from a different angle. This gives you a completely different perspective and can help to move you past stuck, old ways of thinking. Not to mention, it's fun to look at the world from a different perspective! I like to remember my childhood when I attempt this posture. It makes me feel free to take risks and gives me a sense of adventure to approach life from an unusual vantage point.

The lymphatic system greatly benefits from Sirsasana. It enhances a healthy immune system. Since the lymph system has no central pump, lymph is circulated by movement of the musculo-skeletal system, similar to the venous system. This means that through movement as in asana, we support our lymph system. Healthy lymphatic vessels equipped with one-way valves ensure an upward movement of lymph through the body. The Headstand, and body inversions in general, encourages the return of lymph from the lower extremities.

Sirsasana rests the heart and aids circulation, helping to make the body breathe more deeply, oxygenating the blood at a much deeper rate.

Ideally we hold this pose for at least three minutes. This is approximately how long it takes the blood to make one trip through the entire body. Most importantly, however, is to hold this posture only as long as it is comfortable for you.

Cautions

This pose is not suggested for those who have had recent upper body surgery, eye, ear, dental, and so on. In addition, pregnant women should not practice it after the first trimester of pregnancy.

If you have known uncontrolled high blood pressure, diabetes retinopathy, carotid artery disease, glaucoma, or neck problems, please check with a health practitioner before doing this practice. It is wise to concentrate on asanas, which may rectify the condition before you approach the Headstand Pose.

Also, if you are experiencing sinus difficulty with a cold or allergies, it is best to wait until this condition is cleared up before you attempt Headstand Pose so as not to increase the pressure in your sinus cavity. You may experience such discomfort as headaches and eye, ear, and sinus pressure if you practice this pose while having sinus and upper respiratory problems.

Be aware of any dizziness, lightheadedness, or discomfort. At the first sign of any of these, come out of the pose immediately and rest in Savasana.

Real Life

The story you are about to read is one of the most significant examples of real-life success I have ever witnessed personally. This is Reggie's story of transformation through dedication and love for himself and for yoga. This was his wake-up call to enlightenment, and I encourage and support him on his journey. May you, too, be encouraged and supported in your daily life and practice.

"In 1965 I bought a little book written by an Indian yogi and taught myself some basic yoga postures. I did not know anyone who did yoga and so I just practiced on my own. Even in those days my favorite pose was the Headstand ...

Now picture a 375-pound, 56-year-old man who went to the movies and could barely fit into his seat. I couldn't even walk up and down the steps in the theatre without losing my balance!

I started a regular yoga practice almost exactly two years ago. I was desperate for something to help me with a massive weight problem and multiple health problems. The doctors thought that I might have a blocked artery and they were going to do surgery if needed. My feet were completely numb from diabetes and I was taking four strong doses of Neurontin every day for peripheral neuropathy.

To top off my physical condition, I was just flat-out angry and had a terrible case of road rage. In other words, I was a mess and a disaster waiting to happen. I had to do something for myself, and quickly!

So how was I going to get back into yoga? The universe just seemed to open up for me when I decided that I would take up yoga again. One day I walked into Wild Oats Market and there was this lady doing chair massage. In those days my neck hurt all the time so I decided to get a massage. We talked some and she told me she was a yoga instructor. I told her I had decided to take up yoga as a practice and she cheerfully invited me to a class.

I went to the class several nights later and Bliss, my instructor, was very kind and helpful to me. I needed the kindness because I was painfully aware that I was very heavy and very inflexible. Forget the Headstand, I could not even put my legs together when I lay on my back to bring my knees up to my chest.

I know I was on edge, because at one point Bliss had us do the Supine Bound Angle Pose and said this was a surrendering position and that we might feel some emotions. Well, I just cried and cried all through Savasana.

I e-mailed Bliss and told her what happened. She e-mailed back to me and said it was a normal response to opening our hearts and this made me feel better. So I kept going to class because I knew she was a special kind of person and yoga teacher.

I was taking classes with Bliss and I also started taking a class at the YMCA three times per week at seven in the morning. Two months later and I was taking yoga classes almost every day. I lost about 60 pounds in 6 months and was beginning to think about actually trying the Headstand.

I think instinctively I decided that yoga might heal me and help me lose the massive amount of weight. When I thought about yoga I naturally thought about the Headstand, which was discouraging since doing a headstand at 375 pounds would injure my neck. So, the Headstand Pose became a symbol of what I wanted to achieve. When I did one again for the first time in many years, it was, in a word, *priceless*.

During Bliss's class, I asked her to help me with a wall-supported headstand and with her support I was up and fulfilling my dream. I was so gratified.

Since that day I have done yoga and included the Headstand Pose almost every time. I can now do the pose for the length of 25 long strong breaths. In yoga we count length of poses by breaths and not by time. I do this 25-breath Headstand most of the time when I do an asana session, and that's at least once per day and sometimes twice per day. I look forward to the Headstand perhaps more than any other pose because I know when I do it I am going to feel free and clear, not only while I am in the pose but for the rest of the day.

I now have lost 115 pounds and all my medical parameters are normal. My diabetes is gone and I no longer take medication for peripheral neuropathy, and I have full feeling and use of my feet. My blood pressure went from 160/100 to within normal limits and my cholesterol is now 190 from 310. I am living a completely different life from two years ago.

By the way, I still take class with Bliss every chance I get because her classes are a total meditation and relaxation, and she takes beginners like me and builds strength and confidence in them to the point where they can go where their dreams take them."

(Reggie continues to integrate his yoga practice into his life. He accomplished much physically, emotionally, and mentally but not without dedication, discipline, and love for himself, which expands outwardly to others. He is a living example of how yoga can so richly empower our lives.)

Empowerment Journal

As I was writing this book, I asked the students in my classes if they would be interested in contributing their stories of how yoga has affected them. The response was overwhelmingly positive and I marvel at every one of these transformational stories that they shared with me.

Learn what you are and be such.
—Pindar, Greek poet

Here is Judith's story:

As long as I have been working I have been bothered with tightness, spasms, and knots in my neck, back, and shoulders. As I took on more responsibilities in my job, the stress has become worse. My massage therapist used to wince whenever I called for an appointment. The problem was exacerbated after I lifted a piece of luggage from a conveyor belt at the airport and pulled a muscle that ran from my neck to shoulder blade. I was suffering so badly I saw a sports medicine physician who prescribed weeks of physical therapy. I was ready to make the first appointment when a friend of mine asked me to go to yoga classes with her.

Fortunately for me, I accepted her invitation. Through yoga I have managed to keep my neck, back, and shoulder problems under control. I no longer go to bed in pain at night only to wake up the next morning still in pain. My sister asked me what I was doing differently because she noticed my posture had improved so much.

I now live a more enjoyable life in which I don't grunt or moan every time I get up from a chair. I can trim my own toenails, wash my own back, and zip my own dress. Most importantly, I am living a life of true peace.

Mantras for Daily Living

By now, mantras should be a regular part of your yoga practice, which you easily integrate into your daily life. Have you noticed a difference in your perceptions as you repeat a mantra? Can you feel the subtle shifts that occur within your body, mind, and emotions as you concentrate on what you are repeating?

> Happiness lies in the fulfillment of the spirit through the body.
> —Cyril Connolly, English essayist, critic, and novelist

Following are examples of mantras that empower us to become a fully alive person, to enjoy life, and to release old hurts from the past. As we experience the present moments of our life and stop worrying about the past and future, which we cannot live in anyway, we will feel everything in the present from joy to sorrow. The fact is, we will live in empowerment because we can experience all of our thoughts, emotions, and physical sensations honestly and truthfully. There is no other place for living but in the present moment.

For today, pick your favorite mantra from this list or make up your own and recite it first during your yoga or meditation practice and then throughout the day when you think of it. At the end of the day, check in with yourself to see how you feel. Has your mantra helped you to focus? Do you feel more joyful and connected to the present moment? Take some time to really feel the changes that have occurred within you.

- "I can achieve everything through love."
- "Play, play, play!"
- "This too shall pass."
- "I trust the whisper of my inner voice."
- "I release and forgive the past."
- "Joy fills my life."

Transcending Your Practice to Become the Self

Transcendence is the act of going beyond ordinary limits in our thoughts and beliefs. It is moving to the deeper dimension of our Self. In this deeper dimension, we realize that we are much more than the physical body we inhabit and we far surpass the thoughts and emotions we experience in our human form. However, transcending past our ordinary limits is not easily accomplished and requires practice, dedication, and the desire to reach enlightenment.

There is no purifier like knowledge in this world: time makes man find himself in his heart.
—The *Bhagavad-Gita*

Throughout the chapters of this book, we have learned to empower our life by recognizing and following our dharma, our life path, through the spiritual practices of our sadhana. Empowerment comes to us through commitment and service to our self and others and especially in the realization of impermanence. Nothing stays the same, and therefore, letting go of expectations, past slights, and future fears will release us from attachment and enable us to live fully.

Thanks to Patanjali and the Eight-Limbed Path of Ashtanga Yoga, we have a guide to help us empower our life so that we may achieve transcendence from this earthly consciousness to the awakened state of unconditional love. Through yoga, meditation, and pranayama practice, we begin to apply the principles of a transcendent Self to our entire life. Once we establish our practice and become one with it, there is no separation between it and our life. In essence, our life becomes our practice and we continue to expand our awareness beyond our physical life and into the realm of Spirit.

It is through Spirit that we recognize our divine connection. May we find and experience this connection through unconditional love for our self and for all beings so that we may all know our true Self.

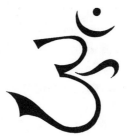

Appendix A

Sanskrit Glossary

Adho Mukha Svanasana   Downward Facing Dog Pose.

Ahimsa   Non-violence; abstention from harmful actions, thoughts, and words toward self and others. One of the five moral principles or "yamas" from the Yoga Sutras.

Anjali mudra   Prayer hand gesture, the "seal of honoring."

Aparigraha   Greedlessness or non-grasping.

Ardha Matsyendrasana   Half Spinal Twist.

Asana   A yoga posture or pose.

Ashtanga Yoga   Eight-limbed union, the eight-fold yoga of Patanjali consisting of moral discipline, self-restraint, posture, breath control, sensory inhibition, concentration, meditation, and ecstasy leading to liberation.

Asteya   Non-stealing.

Baddha Konasana   Bound Angle Pose or Cobbler Pose.

Bandha   Energy lock to create focus and power in the physical and energetic bodies.

Bhagavad-Gita   "The Lord's Song," the oldest and most popular sacred yogic text containing the teachings of Lord Krishna to Arjuna.

Brahmacharya   The practice of chastity in thought, word, and deed. Purity, restraint of sexual energy, one of the five moral observances.

Buddha   Title of Guatama, the founder of Buddhism.

Buddhism   An Eastern religion founded by Buddha based on the premise that "life is suffering."

Chakras   Meaning "wheel," the seven psychoenergetic centers of the body that control the life force energies.

Citta   Consciousness, the finite mind or psyche.

Dharana   Concentration, the sixth limb of the Yoga Sutras.

Dharma   The cosmic law of order, virtue, responsibility, honor.

Dhyana   Meditation or contemplation, the seventh limb of the Yoga Sutras.

Ha   The sun.

Hatha   Forceful, physical.

Hatha Yoga   "Yoga of force." The yoga of physical discipline, aimed at awakening kundalini in the body.

Ishvar-Pranidhana   "Devotion to the Lord." One of the practices of restraining (niyama) in the Yoga Sutras.

Jalandhara Bandha   Throat lock. A technique in Hatha Yoga for confining the life force in the area of the throat.

Jnana mudra   Wisdom hand gesture, "wisdom seal," thumb and forefinger come together on each hand.

Karma   Action or activity of any kind that is done in service for others or self. It is sometimes referred to the concept of cause and effect.

Karma Yoga   The yoga of action or the yoga of service.

Kundalini   "Coiled one," the serpent power that lies dormant in the lowest chakra of the body. Upon its awakening it rises to the seventh chakra to bring identification with the Self.

Kundalini Yoga   The innermost teaching of Hatha Yoga focusing on liberation.

Mahabharata   One of India's two great national epics, recounting the great war between the Kauravas and Pandavas. The epic contains many instructional passages, including the *Bhagavad-Gita*.

Mantra   A sacred sound that empowers the mind for concentration and the transcendence of ordinary states of consciousness.

Meditation   Contemplation or deepening of concentration.

Metta   Loving kindness meditation.

Mudra   "Seal," hand gesture or bodily posture which has symbolic significance but is also thought to conduct the life energy in the body in specific ways.

Nadi Shodhana   "The sweet breath," conduit or channel. A form of alternate nostril breathing.

Namasté   Greeting: "I honor you as I honor myself. I acknowledge we are all *One*."

Nataraja   Sanskrit term for King (or Lord) of the Dance. "Nata" translates to "dancer"; "Raja" translates to "king."

Natarajasana   Dancing Shiva Pose; also known as King of the Dance Pose.

Navasana   Boat Pose.

Niyama   Restraint, the second limb of the Yoga Sutras, which consists of the practice of purity, contentment, austerity, study, and devotion to the Lord.

Om   A divine mantra chanted during meditation that symbolizes the absolute, the primordial sound of the Universe.

Om Mani Padme Hum   "The jewel of consciousness is in the heart's lotus." This mantra emphasizes that anything is possible when the heart and mind are connected. It is the most commonly recited mantra in the world.

Padmasana   Lotus Pose.

Paramahansa Yogananda (d. 1952)   The first yoga master of India whose mission was to live and teach in the West; author of *Autobiography of a Yogi*.

Parvatasana   Seated Mountain Pose.

Paschimotanasana   Stretch of the West Side Pose.

Patanjali   Author of the Yoga Sutras, the source text of classical yoga.

Prana   Life, the life force sustaining the body. Breath is the external manifestation of the life force.

Pranayama   Breath control, the careful regulation of breath, which is the fourth limb of the Yoga Sutras.

Pratyahara   Withdrawal, the fifth limb of the Yoga Sutras; it refers to sensory withdrawal.

The Rig Veda   Oldest sacred Hindu texts.

Sadhana   "Realizing," the path to spiritual realization, a particular practice to reach enlightenment.

Samadhi   "Ecstasy," supraconscious ecstasy that is free from all thought.

Samtosha   Contentment.

Sanskrit   The oldest extant Indo-Aryan language, retained in India in a classical form of language of literature.

Sat Nam   "I am truth."

Satya   Truthfulness.

Savasana   Corpse Pose.

Setu Bandasana   Bridge Pose.

Shanti   Peace.

Shauca   Purity.

Siddhasana   Perfected Being Pose or Perfect Pose.

Sirsasana   Headstand Pose.

Sitali pranayama   Cooling Breath.

Svadhyaya   Self-study.

Tadasana   Mountain Pose.

Tapas   Term for austerity; the literal meaning is heat or to glow.

Tha   Moon.

Tratak   Steady gazing (open eye meditation).

Trikonasana   Triangle Pose.

Ujjayi Breath   Pranayama that is performed by inhaling through both nostrils and drawing the breath down the throat and deeply into the lungs while using the throat lock (Jalandhara Bandha). This produces a resonant sound in the throat.

Upanishads   "Sitting near," Vedic scriptures, sacred texts.

Urdhva Mukha Svanasana   Upward Facing Dog Pose.

Ustrasana   Camel Pose.

Uttanasana   Standing Forward Bend Pose.

Vajrasana   Firm Pose.

Virabhadrasana   Warrior Pose.

Vedas   Ancient Hindu scriptures.

Vritti   Scattered thoughts.

Vrkasana   Tree Pose.

Yamas   Discipline, first limb of the Yoga Sutras comprising the five moral observances (also known as the Hindu god of death).

Yoga   Union, to yoke, practice of balancing energies of the body, mind, and spirit.

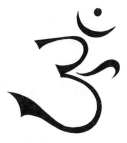

Appendix B

Resources

I have listed a collection of books, magazines, CDs, videos, music, and websites that you might find helpful as you apply yoga to your life. These suggestions are only a small sampling of the wonderful media available to us as yoga practitioners. May this list be helpful to you and offer a place from which you can expand your practice.

Namasté!

Books

Bhagavad-Gita (many different translations available). This text is the earliest and most popular Yoga scripture containing the teachings of Lord Krishna to Arjuna.

Meditation: The First and Last Freedom. Osho International Foundation, 1996. This is an all-encompassing book on meditation. It covers everything from the definition of meditation to specific methods and guidelines of the practice. There are many types of meditation to choose from, which are explained in detail for the reader.

Budilovsky, Joan, and Eve Adamson. *The Complete Idiot's Guide to Yoga*. Alpha Books, 2001. For the beginning yoga practitioner, this book offers a huge amount of information that is easy to understand. The directions are easy to follow and very user friendly.

Cope, Stephen. *Yoga and the Quest for the True Self*. Bantam Books, 1999. If deepening your spirituality through yoga practice is your goal, this book is a must read. It's like reading a modern-day novel on the ancient practice of yoga.

Feuerstein, Georg. *The Deeper Dimension of Yoga (Theory and Practice)*. Shambhala Publications, Inc., 2003. For the yoga enthusiast, this book not only discusses the practice of Hatha Yoga but explains the philosophies, principles and different styles of yoga. This is an excellent reference.

Judith, Anodea, Ph.D. *Wheels of Life*. Llewellyn Publications, 2002. For information on the chakras, this book is one of the best. There is a large amount of information, which is easy to comprehend and apply.

Lasater, Judith, Ph.D. *Relax & Renew (Restful Yoga for Stressful Times)*. Rodmell Press, 1995. An excellent offering of restorative yoga postures, this book not only speaks to the beginning student but also addresses the needs of female students.

Magazines

Body & Soul
Spirituality & Health
Yoga International
Yoga Journal

CDs and Videos

Kundalini Yoga with Gurmukh. Living Arts, 2000. Awaken your spirit, energize your body, and relax your mind with this invigorating practice.

This video is a vigorous workout and beginning students are cautioned to practice at their own pace.

Power Yoga for Beginners with Rodney Yee. Living Arts, 1998. If you're looking for a good beginning workout, this is the video for you. Encompassing a full workout in 20 minutes, this practice strengthens, energizes, and centers you.

YOGA for Deep Relaxation. Bliss Wood, 2002; independent release, www.just4bliss.com. This is an easy-to-follow Hatha Yoga practice designed and instructed by Bliss Wood. Soothing piano music by Donna Michael sets the mood for this deeply relaxing yoga practice. This is a great audio CD for beginners as well as advanced students who are looking for more from yoga than just a physical workout.

Music

Dewachen (Land of Bliss). Kirby Shelstad, 1998; Love Circle Music, www.kirbyshelstad.com. This mix of Asian and fusion music will transport you to another world as you open your heart to your yoga practice.

Somewhere in the Silence. Donna Michael, 2000; Quarterlight Productions, www.donnamichael.com. A beautiful piano solo to invoke deep relaxation and a sense of total serenity. This CD is a must for any restorative yoga practice.

Transformations. E.J. Cryan, 2000; Inspiring Snow Records, www.inspiringsnow.com. For a more flowing practice, this music will transform your yoga workout to a dance and inspire your own creativity.

Websites

www.ByRegion.net. This site has listings of yoga studios, teachers, and gear that are available all over the United States. Just click on your city and state to find the teachers in your area.

www.just4bliss.com. Bliss Wood's website has information on local classes and national/international workshops that are available. There is also inspirational and practical yoga wisdom that can be applied to daily life.

www.yogafinder.com. A wonderful yoga directory, this website can help you find a class or retreat. It even has a great selection of yoga gear and products.

www.yogafish.com. YogaFish is an online yoga toolbox, bursting with the techniques, sequencing, reviews, and great articles from the yoga world. This is a great site as well to inspire yoga students and teachers to take their practice and their teaching to the next level.

www.yogajournal.com. Like the magazine, this website is full of helpful information on yoga from the most basic questions regarding posture to more in-depth spiritual concepts such as concentration, meditation, and liberation.

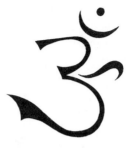

Index